Moral Agendas for Children's Welfare

T0175858

Moral outpourings over what children get up to and the dreadful things that adults do to children are part of the daily diet that is fed to us by newspapers and the broadcasting media. *Moral Agendas for Children's Welfare* goes behind the sensational headlines to question the meaning of morality and moral responsibility towards children in today's society.

By raising uncomfortable questions about the moral justifications for current social practices, such as male circumcision, restrictions on child sexual activities and the exclusion of children from school, this book discusses the problems of how to improve the way that social institutions deal with children so as to make them more responsive to moral principles and judgements on their performance.

Moral Agendas for Children's Welfare addresses the key issue: what is morality and how can it be translated into guiding principles for children's welfare? It will be essential reading for those studying social policy, social work or undertaking socio-legal studies.

Michael King is Professor in the Department of Law and Co-Director of the Centre for the Study of Law, the Child and the Family at Brunel University, Uxbridge.

Moral Agendas for Children's Welfare

Edited by Michael King

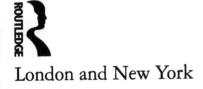

London and New York

First published 1999
by Routledge
11 New Fetter Lane, London EC4P 4EE

Transferred to Digital Printing 2004

Simultaneously published in the USA and Canada
by Routledge
29 West 35th Street, New York, NY 10001

© 1999 Michael King, selection and editorial matter;
individual chapters, the contributors

Typeset in Garamond by Routledge

British Library Cataloguing in Publication Data
A catalogue record for this book is available from the British
Library

Library of Congress Cataloging in Publication Data
Moral agendas for children's welfare / edited by Michael King.
Includes bibliographical references and index.
1. Child welfare–Moral and ethical aspects.
I. King, Michael, 1942–
HV715.M65 1999
362.7–dc21
98–27632
CIP

ISBN 0–415–18012–0 (hbk)
ISBN 0–415–18013–9 (pbk)

Contents

Contributors

David Archard Department of Moral Philosophy, University of St Andrews, Scotland.

Terry Carney School of Law, The University of Sydney, Australia.

Andrew Cooper The Tavistock Clinic, London.

Marinos Diamantides Lecturer, Law Department, Birkbeck College, University of London.

Alison Diduck Centre for the Study of Law, the Child and the Family, Brunel University, Uxbridge.

Stephen Frosh Psychology Department, Birkbeck College, University of London, and The Tavistock Clinic, London.

Ilan Katz National Society for the Prevention of Cruelty to Children, London.

Michael King Centre for the Study of Law, the Child and the Family, Law Department, Brunel University, Uxbridge.

Gillian Miles Child and Family Department, The Tavistock Clinic, London.

Daniel Monk Law Department, Keele University.

Christine Piper Centre for the Study of Law, the Child and the Family, Law Department, Brunel University, Uxbridge.

Rex Stainton Rogers Psychology Department, University of Reading.

Wendy Stainton Rogers School of Health and Social Welfare, Open University, Milton Keynes.

Judith Trowell Child and Family Department, The Tavistock Clinic, London.

Acknowledgements

This book began its life as a workshop on *Moral Agendas for Children's Welfare in the Nineties*, which took place at The Tavistock Centre over two days in July 1996. I should like to thank Judith Trowell for her help in organizing the event. I am also very grateful to the Law Department of Brunel University for their financial contribution towards the workshop, and to The Tavistock Centre for making their facilities available. Finally, my thanks to all those who participated in the workshop, including those who, for one reason or another, have not contributed to the book.

Michael King

1 Introduction

Michael King

What is the point of bringing out a book on children and morality at a time when so many different people already claim to know what is good and bad for children? Ask the editors of tabloid newspapers. They know, as they scream out their knowledge in their reports of the latest paedophile scandal. Ask the Home Secretary. He knows, as he announces yet more measures to punish juvenile offenders and make parents accept responsibility for their children's crimes. Ask those lawyers who represent children in court. They know as they campaign for more rights for children and for more notice to be taken of what children want. Ask social workers, guardians *ad litem* and child psychiatrists – the experts in child abuse. They know what harms children, whether smacking them is good or bad. As they write their reports and make their recommendations, they know with whom children should live, and if and how often they should see their parents. Ask the educationalists. They know, as they set out to identify in the National School Curriculum, what is essential spiritual and moral knowledge for every child at every age. They know that morality can be taught and learnt like any other subject so that every child will, like themselves, know the difference between right and wrong.[1] When these children, these students of morality become parents they will know what is good and bad for their own children, and so we will evolve into more moral beings and the world will become a more moral place.

With so much moral knowledge around in the media, books, videos, CD-ROMS, the Internet, anyone with a few hours to spare can find out all they need about the right and the wrong way to treat children in every imaginable situation. In today's world, morality has become a commodity like any other. If you do not already have it, it is something you can acquire by going through the proper channels, by making the necessary commitment, by doing a course on it, by watching a video about it, by knowing the right people to give you the right answers. Moral mazes may exist, but their existence confirms that there are those who know their way through the maze and all we have to do is ask them for directions.

If this brief account of society's ability to deal with moral issues concerning children appears comforting and reassuring, it might be wise to stop reading at this point, for much of the remainder of the book should perhaps carry a warning that it could seriously damage your peace of mind. *Moral Agendas for Children's Welfare* brings together contributors from different disciplinary backgrounds who share in common an ability to raise disturbing questions about many of our current ideas, beliefs, values and assumptions in relation to children and what is good and bad for them. But this is not all. Several of the chapters in this book do not merely question whether we 'have got things right' or are 'on the right path'. More fundamentally, taken together, they raise the issue as to whether there can be in today's society any notion of notion of absolute right or absolute wrong for children, whether it is even possible to answer questions on morality with the confidence that there is only one correct answer.

Morals and moralizing

Moralizing has never been a more popular activity. In previous times, it was confined largely to gravely intoned sermons from the pulpit or campaigns to save souls from perdition. Today's moralizers are everywhere and there is today no greater attraction to moralizers than anxieties concerning children, their safety, their delinquent or anti-social behaviour, their drug-taking, their sexuality, their health, their education and their general well-being. Yet all this moralizing about children has to be seen in the context of a social world where the terms 'morals' and 'morality' are freely and openly tossed around as if everyone knew exactly what they meant by them. Everyone seems to know what morality is and where to find it. It is also a world where the image that society presents to itself is one of continual improvement. If life is squalid and unhappy for some people or if there are those who behave badly, causing misery and suffering for others, this can be improved simply by turning individuals into better people, people who give to charity, who do not resort to violence, who are not prejudiced or use politically incorrect language.

This instantaneous formulation and mass communication of moral lessons in today's world has become a relatively effortless task. It has never been easier to get masses of people thinking about morality as part of their daily routine. Newspaper editors, politicians, media pundits are engaged in a continual pursuit of stories with *a moral slant*. Their words are picked up by eager ears and read by eager eyes. At no time in history can there have been so much talk of morality. A young woman speaks out to the press and by the next day the vices (and virtues) of the president of the United States have become the talking point not just of the nation, but of the whole world. There are experts to pronounce on the legal position, the political implications, the effect on foreign relations, on the stock market. They speculate on whether he did it or didn't do it, whether he is lying or she is lying, whether it matters or does not matter. The word of a man in high office, his alleged abuse of power, is pitted against that of a slighted woman for everyone to enjoy and engage in congratulating themselves on the moral nature of a society that does so much moralizing.

Yet the source of much of today's global moralizing is not amusement at the president's indiscretions, but anxiety: the phenomenon of society giving itself a fright and then seeking ways of reassuring itself that things are not quite as bad as they first appeared. This creation of a moral crisis in itself may not be an entirely new phenomenon. Anxiety has often in the past been used by politicians rhetorically as a prelude to action against an internal or external enemy. What is different about today's rhetoric of anxiety is its independence from the possibility of immediate solutions for alleviating the anxiety, such as defeating the enemy. So while moralizing and 'the new style of morality' may be 'based on a common interest in the alleviation of anxiety' (Luhmann, 1989, p. 127) it also feeds on the resilience of anxiety. Anxiety over crime continues despite the locking up of more and more criminals and the introduction of strong preventative measures. Concern over global warming continues despite a reduction in the use of CFCs. Saddam Hussein is still a threat, despite his defeat in the Gulf War. Is beef really safe to eat? Children are still 'at risk' of sexual abuse despite anti-paedophile legislation. Even if law, politics and science are able in practice to reduce some of the threats of disease, war, ecological disaster or child abuse, they still find themselves powerless to control anxiety itself. Indeed, attempts at reassurance sound thinner and thinner with each repetition and may themselves have the paradoxical effect of giving rise to further and more widespread anxiety.

Moralizing, on the other hand, has no need immediate need of practical solutions. It is a way of presenting society to itself which brings into the present the comforting reassurances that are supposed to have helped in the past, while offering some hope of a better or safer future. Moralizing in no way holds the moralizers responsible for bringing that desired future into existence. At the same time moralizing puts pressure on society's coping (or function) systems of law, politics and science to come up with solutions. Viewed from the standpoint of morality, therefore, moral principles appear to enter these systems as guiding lights for all future action and, as such, provide a stick for observers to beat the transgressors of these moral principles for their failure to live up to the expectations that the principles demand. In this way, failures to alleviate the causes of anxiety may be attributed to incompetence, negligence, corruption or immorality, which may be rectified by an assertion or reassertion of ethical values to guide the operations of these systems and to restore society's trust in them.

All this presupposes the possibility of adapting morality in ways which take on board a vision of a modern society that is functionally fragmented, as opposed to the vision of a unified and undifferentiated social system in which morality, like God or love or money, is all-pervasive and moves spirit-like directly into every sphere of personal and social existence. While it is true that the rhetoric of morality, the moralizing, may remain within this undifferentiated conceptual world, the practical task of getting people and society to take morality seriously obliges moralizers to face up to a society where the scope for moralizing may be boundless, but the possibilities for moral action may be extremely limited.

How then are moralizers to promote and encourage the creation of *a good society*? The idea, born from religious thought, that a good or moral society may be brought about by making *people* good and moral requires some critical re-examination in the light of a contemporary social organization which systematically separates the private from the public, the social from the interpersonal. The opposite, Marxian, idea that 'it is not the consciousness of men that determines their being, but, on the contrary, their social being that determines their consciousness'[2] is no less in need of critical reappraisal, in the face of psychoanalytical and socio-biological claims that the unconscious or genetic inheritance may be more important than society in determining consciousness. To observe people as a project of society, or society as a projection of people's consciousness risks ignoring a whole range of possibilities that lie on either side of the people/society distinction. By collapsing this distinction and claiming, along with a recent political heroine, that there is no such thing as society, we arrive very close to a Rousseauesque romanticism, a social contract where being moral becomes a self-denying ordinance, an overbearing super-ego. In this way the moral rectitude of a society (assuming such a thing exists) may be judged by observing the behaviour of its individual members. Morality here has the unique task of making judgements about people and their behaviour, of fashioning and destroying reputations. Or putting the cart before the horse, 'there are no good or bad people, but only the possibility of indicating people as good or bad'.[3]

This way of conceptualizing morality as a matter of individual choice and control ignores, however, European and American sociological thought, in the tradition of Durkheim and Weber, which presents the social environment as separate and distinct from individual consciousness. This same distinction, but now framed in terms of culture, also permeates a powerful social anthropological tradition, in which morality becomes part of a cultural inheritance passed on and preserved not, or not only, by individuals, but through the values inherent in social institutions. If, as these traditions urge, we recognize that the environment in which people work, form relationships, take their pleasures and, in complex ways, formulate an identity for themselves and for others, is more than a product of individual or collective invention to be reproduced and reinvented with each new generation, we will have accepted the existence of a separate entity which we may call 'society'. Morality now finds itself situated, not in individual consciousness, or self-denial, but in the norms, values and traditions of societies or cultures.

Communicating morality

A recent theoretical attempt to reconcile these different ways of conceptualizing the moral, while maintaining distinct, yet interdependent notions of people and society has been the notion of *communicative systems*. According to this model, people and society become mediums for each other's communications. This is to propose that those communications which emerge from social systems such as law, politics, science, education, economics, etc. are different in kind from the communications that take place either within the heads of people, their stream of consciousness and internal dialogue, or between people at the level of the intimate or interpersonal.

In the hands of some theorists, the social systems of law, politics, economics and technology become symbols of an immoral order, driven by the self-serving interests of power and money to annihilate the capacity for moral judgements and moral actions which can be found in the 'ideal speech patterns' of the lifeworld of ordinary people in conditions of true democracy.[4] The challenge for modern society, according to this view, is how to reassert true democratic values and give ordinary people a voice in their own lives. These are theories of communication which clearly contain their own distinctive moral agenda, while at the same time recognizing the complexity of modern society and the distinction between the people and those social systems which, they claim, oppress them.

Autopoietic theory, in its account of self-referring communicative systems,[5] on the other hand, offers no clear moral agenda in its rather different view of communicative systems. It recognizes people as necessary for society's existence, just as society is necessary for people's existence. Morality here is not to be found in the ideal speech patterns of ordinary people, emerging spontaneously from their interpersonal relationships. Rather, it is a unique, distinctive way of communicating and so making sense of the phenomenal world by coding that world according to a binary distinction of good/bad, virtue/evil or moral/immoral. Any event or item of information may be reproduced as a moral communication, but, as we shall see, in practice such communications are used to esteem or disesteem people.

According to autopoietic theory, society is seen as the totality of all communications, that is of everything that can be understood as being meaningful. As such it relies upon the continuing operations of *social function systems*, that is those systems which enable the very notion of society to have meaning by providing the impressions of security and stability upon which society depends.[6] These systems include law, science, politics, health economics and education. In past eras the concept of society as a product of divine will, and so subject in all its parts to God's law, made it possible for moral values to be identical or almost identical to the values of these function systems. Criminals, for example were invariably sinners. The rich could see themselves and be seen as favoured because of their inherent virtue; sickness could be linked to wickedness; the monarch, appointed by God, could do no wrong; and scientific discoveries which denied God's version of the world were bad science, as Galileo found to his cost.

In modern society, however, the values of social function systems operate independently of morality. The relation between the moral code and each of these systems is one of contingency rather than mutuality. We are not obliged to condemn a person as immoral simply because he or she loses a court case; falling ill is no longer seen to be a punishment for having sinned; exam failure or being declared redundant are not moral disasters; and political parties do not lose elections because they are morally superior to the winners. Moral judgements may or may not be applied after the event, but the event as communicated by each of these social systems does not itself carry a signifier which has to be interpreted in terms of particular moral values. It could fall on either side of the moral divide, on both sides simultaneously, according to the judgements of different moralizers, or be ignored entirely, being seen as a matter on which moral judgements are not appropriate. Even condemned criminals may be seen as morally justified in their illegal acts or may be regarded as having committed a technical offence only.

Socially functional communications – laws, legal judgements, administrative decisions, share prices, scientific theories, medical diagnoses, exam marks, election results, the issue of certificates of nationality, declarations of war, pronouncements of births, deaths or marriage, the recognition of works of art, etc. – are produced independently of morality through the recursive and repetitive operation of social function systems. These systems are not in any sense of the term moral organizations. On the other hand, it is not feasible for them to ignore entirely the existence of a system of morality within their environment and the possibility that their communications may subsequently be subjected to moral evaluation. While morality may not infiltrate the system's programmes it is, however, capable of undermining society's trust in the system's operations and can raise fundamental questions as to whether any reliance can be placed upon that system's communications. In performing this service moralizers are able to draw attention to fears and anxieties which they themselves have helped to construct and then, as we have seen, offer cosy reassurances from the past concerning the right strategies for reasserting the moral order and restoring trust in the system. Since these moral judgements are directed at people within systems rather than the operations of systems which are too complex and too impersonal for the attribution of moral values, the effects of such moralizing upon the future of society are likely to be extremely limited. But these are matters which require fuller discussion.

The uncertainty of morality

But how do we know what should be seen as moral and what immoral in all of this? Those who see today's society as 'postmodern' point to what they see as the fragmentation and dislocation not only of society, but also of each individual's subjective identity within that society. What was a unified whole is now 'a life in fragments',[7] and a divided and fractured world characterized by the absence of certainties and the failure of grand theories (including religion) that were once able to provide these certainties. Nobody today can be sure that their conception of right and wrong, of good and evil, will coincide with that of their neighbour or even that their neighbour will share with them the same evaluative framework for making moral judgements. If this level of uncertainty were to pervade all spheres of social existence, there would indeed be some justification in pronouncing the death of modernity and labelling today's society as 'postmodern' (assuming always that society still existed as a community where meaning could be shared!). Nevertheless, more pragmatic and less theoretical observers of today's society have no difficulty in finding certainties – not perhaps the grand certainties of the past about the existence of God or the infallibility of science, but those myriads of 'truths' and 'facts' that allow daily life to continue and decisions to be made. In the phenomenal world where most people live out their daily lives, it is very much business as usual.

While it is certainly true that today's certainties may indeed be tomorrow's fallacies, this has always been the case; all that has changed is the speed with which tomorrow follows today. For those who have to make their way in the real world of the present today's certainties are still certain and have to be treated as such, until such time as they are replaced. What distinguishes modern society from past eras is not its fragmentation and consequent instability – it has not been smashed and stuck together – but the dependence for its stability upon the constant readjustment of highly differentiated systems for observing and making sense of the world – the social function systems that we have already glimpsed. Law, politics, economics, science, religion, the media, etc. operate according to very clearly defined truths and certainties, but their currency, their validity as guides to expectations and understanding, end at their borders. It is not that society is fragmented, but rather that each system constructs a *total* version of society which serves its own purposes and incorporates its own norms and values, and observes the norms and values of other systems from its own limited perspective.

The values of these functional systems are not, as we have noted, identical to moral values. Furthermore, any attempt to substitute a moral code for that of the system could result in uncertainty as to the significance of that system's communications, and eventual loss of faith in the reliability of the system. On occasions, however, the system's outcomes will coincide with those of certain moralizers. Legal decisions may be equitable, condemn discrimination or relieve oppression, but there is nothing in the programme of the legal system that would guarantee this outcome by making a failure to conform with moral values unlawful. If law and justice are but distant cousins, as Alison Diduck tells us in Chapter 8 of this book, there may well be very good reasons for this distant relationship. While the law is what the legal system decides it must be, who can determine what constitutes justice? If judges were to decide from their own individual notions of what is just, there is no guarantee that their decisions would coincide with the judgements of moralizers. Moreover, if they happen to coincide with those of some moralizers, they would almost certainly clash with the values of others. In such a case the certainty and dependability of legal communications for other systems, the very avoidance of the necessity of relying upon an individual's judgement would end abruptly.

In a similar manner, if morality were to determine what happened in other social institutions, financial investments would have to be evaluated on the basis, say, of their ethicality, rather than their profitability; political parties would fight elections on the ground of their moral superiority to the opposition; expensive medical treatment would be offered only to those who merited it; scientific research would be judged by the good or evil purposes to which it could be applied; and first class degrees would be given only to those students who had led virtuous lives. It is clear that, once the organization of society had evolved along the lines of functional differentiation, the withdrawal of morality from social function systems became inevitable, for there was no possibility of combining the moral code of good/bad with the code which allowed the function systems to generate in their communications the reliable information necessary for society to exist.

Similar problems occur when attempts are made to use the moral system as if it were able to operate functionally and produce such communications of estimation and disestimation as are needed for a minimum level of social co-ordination to elicit responses in other social function systems. However unambiguous the message of moralizers may be, there is no guarantee that the positive or negative label will stick. A nun who has devoted her life to the care of the terminally ill may still have detractors who portray her as a self-seeking publicist. On the other side of the distinction, the directors of multinational corporations who systematically destroy the environment, for example, still have admirers among the shareholders who profit from their operations, employees who earn a good living working for these corporations and the governments who gain from their presence in the country. Moralizing alone is unlikely to shame them into making their behaviour more virtuous when virtue itself has more than one face and the exploiters of the earth's resources can simply choose a facet of virtue that justifies and legitimates their operations – the relief of local poverty, for example. Nor are these in any way unique examples.

Indeed, it is difficult to think of a case where the application of one moral principle does not raise one or more counter-principles with no reliable way of resolving which of these conflicting principles should apply. Every issue that moralizing identifies as a moral issue is potentially also a moral dilemma. The evocation of the philosopher heroes of the nineteenth century or from ancient Greece or Rome does not help to resolve such dilemmas today. Nor does recourse to universal human rights as the supreme moral code, for the exercise of one right frequently transgresses another or, at the very least, gives rise to an exception which can be deployed to show why the right should not be exercised in this particular case. Even torture can be justified on the grounds of being the lesser evil.

At the end of the twentieth century, therefore, one does not look to morality for certainties. On the contrary, any attempt to apply the moral code without some additional justification, whether it be economic, medical or legal, is likely to throw open the doors of controversy, and force difficult and often insoluble problems out into the open. Certainties have to be found elsewhere, notably within the boundaries of those communicative systems which have the capacity to reduce or avoid altogether the unstable reliance on faith or experience. Law is the prime example, avoiding the need for moral evaluation, by making the decision of lawful/unlawful a technical task of applying rules to facts. Even deciding whether a wrongful intention accompanied a harmful act has been reduced to a technical exercise by rules assuming *mens rea* or by avoiding the question all together through the imposition of absolute liability. Even the sentencing of those guilty of murder, at least in the United Kingdom, cannot take into account different degrees of blame. Law has no obligation to burden itself with difficult moral questions such as those concerning motivation or free will and determinism. It may either disregard them entirely or, alternatively, transform them into simple rules of thumb. Once moral principles have been transformed into legal rules, they evolve according to law's programmes and not according to morality's. Using legal communications as a guide, society knows for certain who are the guilty and the careless, even where law itself in its internal operations may have been equivocal, as in the case of a majority verdict.

This is not to suggest that law is impervious to changes in moral values. On the contrary, such changes frequently result in shifts in the law, either through the courts or through the intermediary of legislation through the political system. Yet, as we have noted, there is no guarantee that this will happen. The identification of law with moral values may be a favourite pastime of jurisprudential scholars, but it has no validity outside the closed (often utopian) world that they have constructed for themselves – a world that does not exist outside their scholarly endeavours.

Economic programmes also produce certainties which may appear to take on the form of reconstructed morality. Aid from rich to poor nations, for example, may be made dependent upon the poor nation's respect for human rights, but the morality of such an exercise is put in doubt when it becomes clear that it is the sick, the aged and children who are hit hardest by economic sanctions. Stockbrokers may introduce codes of practice and ethics committees in an effort at self-regulation, but this does not prevent people from losing money. The invention of such devices as rewarding charity by public acknowledgement of donations and social esteem for benefactors may give the appearance of wealth and virtue going hand in hand but only as long as nobody thinks of asking how the wealth was acquired in the first place. Moral messages may, of course, be transformed into money, whether in the form of T-shirts to mourn the death of a martyred princess or guided tours of the sites of London's most horrific murders. But these messages do not in any way alter economic programmes. Economic certainties, that losses and gains will be made, that property will be acquired and sold, that prices will go up and down therefore exist quite independently of moral agendas.

In political life, the fact that a politician may have acted immorally does not automatically disqualify him or her from holding office, as we saw at the start of this chapter. As Machiavelli (1532) so shockingly revealed, political values are not entirely congruent with moral values. It is readily accepted, for example, that politicians cannot be trusted to tell the truth about their intentions, or to keep their promises, but this does not make them bad statesmen. Such immorality can readily be justified on the basis of *raisons d'état* or the public interest. On the other hand, politics and morality cannot be kept entirely separate. We expect our politicians not to take bribes, use illegal surveillance techniques or deliberately mislead parliament and the public, for such misconduct undermines the very foundations of politics, just as the taking of drugs undermines sport, and plagiarism undermines education. To this extent politics depends upon moral approval, and where moral disapproval occurs it is likely to take the form of a public scandal and media hounding of those politicians who have stepped out of line.

To summarize, the relation between morality and society's function systems is a complex one. The essential nature of these systems is one of amorality in the sense that the values of these systems are not moral values. At the same time they are not surrounded by an impermeable membrane which protects them entirely from moral communications. In so far as these systems need moral approval to convince society that their communications can be trusted, they are dependent upon morality. Seen from a moral perspective, morality appears like a guard dog which, through the vigilance of the media, keeps the operations of function systems under continual surveillance. The systems are able to some degree to throw morality off the scent by the introduction of self-policing mechanisms such as ethics committees, which give the impression that the moral code has entered the system and is working in harmony with the system's own coding. In practice the two codes are kept entirely separate, and self-policing acts as a net which catches and subjects to moral scrutiny *only some of the system's activities*, while allowing others to pass through as if they were devoid of moral content.

The coincidence that occurs from time to time of a system's values with those of morality, is sufficient to convince moralizers of the possibility of a permanent or long-term coupling between the two codes so that the terms good, moral and virtuous will eventually become congruent with the terms legal, profitable, politically expedient, scientifically true, healthy, academically successful, etc., so that moral agendas may also become legal, political, economic, scientific, medical and educational agendas. Yet, attractive as such projects must appear, they have no chance of success, since under the conditions in which modern society exists there is no possibility of morality controlling function systems, because the internal programmes of law, politics, economics, science, etc. cannot be moralized. All that can be moralized is people, their virtues and their vices, their strengths and their imperfections. The programme of morality is to reproduce and communicate function system failures as individual failings and so allow the normal business of the system to carry on as usual.[8] By emphasizing the importance of individuals, political, financial, scientific or social work scandals are able to create the impression that the moral integrity of the system can be restored by dismissals and resignations. Only people, and never the mechanisms of the system, may be made the subject of moral indignation. This is not to say that, once the excitement has died down, system failures may become the subject of critical scrutiny, but that any examination of these failings will be technical, and not moral, in nature. Even where their starting point is some moral principle, they will inevitably focus on the structures of the system. Any reforms resulting from these critical examinations will most probably take the form of changes in procedure or requirements for more highly or differently qualified decision-makers. Applying these reforms may make the operations of the system quicker, more efficient and more responsive to public demands, but only by seeing virtue as equivalent to efficiency will the system appear to be more moral. In such scandals and their aftermath the limitations of the moral code in modern society and the continuing amorality of social function systems are implicitly acknowledged.

We end this first chapter, therefore, with no more knowledge than we started as to what is morally right or morally wrong for children's welfare. Indeed, this chapter, by implication, challenges the claims of moralizers that they know the answers to moral issues and that they know how to make us or our children more moral. Yet it does not mount a direct challenge to these claims, for it does not say, 'I am right and you are wrong' or 'I know better than you'. Rather it describes the difficulties for moral communications in the modern world – difficulties which not only deprive moral judgements of any universal acceptance or application, but which also limit morality, as a discourse or system of communication, to the world of the interpersonal, of intimate relations, the private rather than the public sphere. This does not mean to say that this interpersonal world does not enter the public arena at all. The daily reports in the press and media of human frailty, whether the corruption of public officials or the love affairs of pop stars, clearly argue against such an interpretation. Through the press and media the public gaze enters the private world of individuals and imposes moral judgements on their behaviour. These moral judgements, however, are contested and controversial. Some may approve; others may disapprove, while others still may question whether the issue should be one for morality in the first place. While making people's private lives public, these reports and the moral judgements they make, remain nevertheless within the sphere of private uncertainty in that they give no clear directions as to how society should respond to them or what precisely it should do about their moral judgements. As we have seen, for these interpersonal communications to become translated into social communications, some action has to be taken by one or more social institutions. Decisions have to be made and these decisions have to be recognized as authoritative. The miscreants may be prosecuted or sued in the civil courts; the victims may be compensated; political heads may roll; major changes in the way that society is ordered may be based on the advice of experts on what should be done and on how to avoid similar occurrences in the future. In this process the moral judgement becomes transformed into something other than morality. Moreover, there is no guarantee that the decisions that are made in the public sphere will make people more (or less) moral.

It would be a mistake to interpret the message from this chapter as advice not to take moralizers too seriously, because their pronouncements are unlikely to affect anything important in our lives. On the contrary, the message is to take moralizers very seriously, because you never know and have no way of knowing what their moral judgements might lead to. With this in mind, let us turn specifically to moral concerns relating to children.

Notes

1 See Schools Curriculum and Assessment Authority (SCAA) (1995, 1996).
2 Karl Marx, *A Contribution to the Critique of Political Economy*, 1959.
3 For further elaboration, see Luhmann (1993a), p. 1000.
4 These terms relate to the theory of communicative action as expounded by Jürgen Habermas. See Habermas (1984, 1987).
5 I am indebted to Niiklas Luhmann's two essays on morality (Luhmann, 1993a and 1994) for his interesting vision of the moral system and its code to which I refer throughout this chapter.
6 In the autopoietic model of modern society, social communications, unlike interpersonal communications, reflect the historic fragmentation of modern society into separate systems, such as law, politics, science, economics, etc. These differ from one another in terms of their functions, rather than their position in a hierarchical or centre-periphery structure of the kind that characterized the organization of past societies. The communications of one system, whether legal decisions, scientific theories, economic forecasts or acts of parliament, can be relied upon to control the communications of any other system, since each system is able to carry on in a self-referential way, producing communications from its own operations. On the other hand, none of these systems can be totally independent of the others, for each relies upon the others to produce information which form part of that system's environment and may well influence its internal operations. See Luhmann (1986, 1995); Teubner (1993); King and Schütz (1994).
7 *Life in Fragments* is the title of Zygmunt Bauman's (1995) critique of modernism in which he welcomes the questioning of fundamental truths and the relativism that it has encouraged. For a more critical view of postmodernism see Gellner (1992), *Postmodernism, Reason and Religion*.
8 See Luhmann (1994), p. 34.

2 Images of children and morality

Michael King

Moral agendas and 'the child'

The title of this book situates agendas, or projects, for the welfare of children in a moral framework. The subject of these agendas is primarily children themselves: how to make them better, purer, more responsible, less selfish, less violent, etc. Of course, the moral status attributed to children at the outset, the images of the child that a parent, school or society have constructed, determines in no small degree the moral agendas which the child is presumed to need.[1] Children as innocents, for instance, need protecting and fostering, while children who are inherently evil require regimes of restraint and improvement.

A second category of moral agenda is directed at those who, through their actions and attitudes, affect children's lives, those who, for example, have the care of children or who, as parents, teachers or in other capacities, regularly take decisions about them or on their behalf. Here again, moral agendas will take as their starting point a particular social construction of 'the child', but also important will be the part that children are seen to be playing in the lives of the adults, and the expectations associated with the adult's relations with the child. They will concentrate not only on the child's needs, but also on the adult's capacity to meet those needs and ways of improving that adult's performance. While some general moral principles clearly exist, such as setting a good example to children, others are associated with particular adult roles, such as mother, father, step-parent, teacher, doctor or police officer.

In both these categories of moral agenda, morality remains at the level of interpersonal relations – the behaviour of the child towards others or the behaviour of others towards that child. There is, however, a third category of moral agenda which increasingly features in the programmes of those who wish to improve children's lives: agendas aimed at social processes and social institutions. These agendas set out images of both children and those responsible for or about to be responsible for their immediate welfare, but, in addition set out the ways in which the institution or process concerned, be it law, politics, medicine, education, big business, the media, may improve children's lives or desist from conduct which is likely to harm them. Moral agendas appear here like lobbyists in the corridors of power, urging those whom they see as able to affect children's well-being to take on board their particular image of the child and/or carer.

In this category of agenda it is not individuals, but social systems which are being unjust to children, damaging the health of children, ruining the lives of children, failing to answer the needs of children, being cruel to children, etc. In Chapter 1 I argued that these systems were 'amoral' in that they did not operate in accordance with a moral code, but always referred back to their own communications rather than to moral principles. This does not, however, prevent others, including some of the contributors to this book, from seeing them as having specific moral agendas and seeking to influence those agendas in ways which they claim will benefit children. While such pursuits may well raise expectations as to the ability of the system to act in moral ways, it seems unlikely that the system will be able to fulfil these expectations, for the reasons set out in Chapter 1. The agenda then becomes one of trying to make the values of the system *coincide with* rather than *adopt* a particular view of morality.

The different chapters of this book present accounts of all three kinds of moral agenda; agendas which both evoke and are constructed around contrasting images of children as in Daniel Monk's account of 'the special needs child' and 'the school excluded child' (Chapter 13); agendas aimed at making children appear more like adults and, therefore more prone to be treated as adults, as Alison Diduck recounts in her chapter (Chapter 8); and moral agendas for the sexual behaviour of children (and of adults towards children) which Wendy and Rex Stainton Rogers demonstrate have been formulated around different images of childhood sexuality (Chapter 11). Marinos Diamantides, alone among the contributors, directs attention specifically at parents and other care-takers and their moral responsibilities towards the children in their care (Chapter 7).

For these and other writers in this volume the objects of attention or concern are not only interpersonal relations, but also social institutions in which implicit or explicit moral agendas determine or influence the rules and processes of the institution, and the decisions that are made on issues of children and their welfare. Some, such as Stephen Frosh (Chapter 12) in his discussion of religious fundamentalism, or Andrew Cooper in his chapter on the courts (Chapter 10) are critical of institutions which blindly follow their own agendas without recognizing the harm that they may be causing to children, or seeing that harm as a lesser evil than disobeying institutional rules. Others, such as Ilan Katz (Chapter 6), recognize that two different institutional agendas, in Katz's case those of religion and child protection, both claiming to be moral, may coexist in modern society without any possibility of knowing which is better (or more moral) than the other.

Contributions to the debate

The recent history of moralizing about children's welfare

Both Christine Piper (Chapter 3) and Terry Carney (Chapter 4) consider, from very different angles, the ways in which moral issues concerning children have historically entered the political, and subsequently legal, arena. Christine Piper's account is that of a social historian. She writes about moral campaigns for children in the nineteenth century, drawing our attention to the difficulties faced by reformers in translating their admirable intentions into laws that were acceptable to politicians who had other things on their mind than children's welfare. In presenting this account, she demonstrates how changes in society alter political perceptions, not only of children and their needs, but also of what is considered to be 'an evil' against which it is legitimate for the government and the courts to act. In the case of campaigns to protect children, it was not simply a matter of evil being 'in the eyes of the beholder', but rather that Victorian society's investment in the image of the father as the figure of authority for the family prevented the formulation of any public moral statements which implicated fathers as sources of evil in relation to their children.

According to Piper, it was this image of the unimpeachable 'father of the family' and the belief that undermining the family was a far greater evil than that of protecting children which prevented the passing of child welfare legislation until the 1880s: 'Once it had become possible to label particular parents as the source of the harm suffered by their child then the way was open for other harms to justify...intervention in the family.' This has paved the way for the present situation at the end of the twentieth century, in which the political agenda in relation to children in dysfunctional or dangerous families wavers unsteadily between supporting parents so that they are better able to fulfil their moral responsibilities towards their children, and blaming them and removing their children when things go wrong. If one wished to contrast today's situation with that of the nineteenth century, one could argue that what makes politicians' lives so much more difficult today is that different moral principles may be invoked by different moral campaigners, be they feminists or family rights advocates, to support diametrically opposite forms of intervention in the lives of children and their families. Moreover, whereas in Victorian times religion and later science could be relied upon at any one time to point a knowledgeable finger at the path to take, with little fear of contradiction, today there seem to be too many paths and no reliable way of deciding which one is the right one to take.

Terry Carney's contribution (Chapter 4) grapples with this very problem. In his hands, it takes the form of a search for the political model which is best able to put into practice moral values concerning children's welfare in modern society. Having reviewed policies towards deprived and delinquent children over the past two centuries, including the demise of the welfare state as originally conceived in the 1940s and 1950s, he turns his attention to recent political theories which attempt to engage individuals in the collective enterprise of constructing a secure world in which children's interests may flourish. He considers the social democratic solution, 'social citizenship' and 'active citizenship', with its emphasis on fostering 'the interests of (young) citizens in participating in the life of the community'. He then moves on to 'contractualism' and the dismantling of state provision in favour of private services, with the state acting as overseer or manager of profit-seeking service providers. Both these solutions, he argues, have their advantages and their disadvantages, but 'more attention needs to be paid to finding ways of further *dissolving* the dichotomy between the public and the private spheres of action'. He goes on to identify two methods of achieving this blend between private and public. One, which he sees as emerging from postmodern scholarship, is that of the 'dialogic community'. It is built on relations of interdependence which may arise outside the law and the traditional boundaries of the state. Yet, without some legal or political framework which guarantee respect and responsibility towards weaker members of society such as children, it is difficult to see how moral values are likely to be established and sustained, unless, of course, one believes in the inherent goodness of human nature. The other way of blending the private and the public, according to Carney, is 'communitarianism'. This solution may be strong in ethical content, with notions of understanding and co-operation being seen as central moral values, but it rests on the fragile foundations of voluntarism and community support, which may not be able to resist the countervailing forces of, for example, individualism and rampant commercialism.

The results of Carney's deliberations from within the arena of political theory could perhaps have been anticipated from the conclusions that Chapter 1 of this book reached in its sociological survey of social function systems: the impossibility of the political system being taken over by moral values. If these values enter the system it is in a form which makes them recognizable as political communications, that is as policies or political solutions to social problems. As such what was once a moral principle is obliged to do business with all those other values and interests that vie for attention within the discourse of politics. It is not perhaps surprising, therefore, that in the last analysis Carney moves away from grand political ideas to more modest proposals, such as family group conferences or other popular justice institutions, which may possibly be able to exist at the level of interpersonal communications without having to win political approval.

The problem of definitions

For observers of social systems the answer to the question whether morality can refer to anything but the behaviour of individuated human beings as the only possible moral agents is clear. Any attempts to make these systems somehow morally responsible always reverts in time back to an issue of individual human failings. For moral philosophers, however, the question is still an open one and, according to David Archard (Chapter 5) is a matter of 'familiar and long-standing debate'. It is a debate which is highly pertinent to the issue of child abuse, which is the subject of Archard's philosophical inquiry. In his chapter he seeks to know whether it is possible to define 'child abuse' in a way that would cover all those forms of morally reprehensible behaviour that are recognized as causing serious harm to children while, at the same time, excluding things that go wrong in children's lives to which we would not wish to attach any moral label. He sets out his requirements for a clear, unambiguous definition of child abuse. For example, 'open texture' terms, such as 'proper', 'normal' or 'adequate', of which the interpretation may be a matter of reasonable disagreement, would have to be avoided, as would categories of harm which imposed 'impossible or unreasonable demands on those charged with the responsibility of caring for a child'.

Archard goes on to consider two different types of definition of

child abuse. First, there is the 'orthodox', which covers those definitions which appear in official documents. Here, abuse is divided into
discrete categories and limited to 'a constrained group of specific,
serious harms', the intention being to identify those children, on
whose behalf some official action should be taken. Second, there exist
'persuasive definitions'. These give 'a new conceptual meaning to a
familiar word without substantially changing its emotive meaning'
(Stevenson, 1938, p. 331). They may be used by people to persuade
others that something not previously covered by the term is child
abuse and should be viewed with the same disapproval that attaches to
all other instances of child abuse. Terms such as 'real', 'genuine' or
'true' often accompany these definitions.

Archard goes on to explain that the definition of child abuse has
been difficult to fix because, first of all, it is of recent origin and its
very newness makes it easier to manipulate than concepts that have a
long-established history, and second, because 'there have been a variety
of interested groups seeking to supply the definitive account of the
phenomenon'. He adds to these problems that of attributing harm to
children on the part of social, economic or political practices, institutions and arrangements. The question, he argues, 'is not whether
significant harms befall children because they live under certain kinds
of social and political arrangements', but rather whether they are
wronged by so living, where the accusation of wrongdoing presupposes
responsibility and the responsibility is laid at the door of the set of
arrangements. In order to make judgements of 'evil regimes' or 'evil
policies', it would be necessary to have consistent criteria which distinguished between those governments who callously and deliberately
exploit and injure children, and those who are inept or misguided and
under whose mismanagement or fanaticism children suffer harm.
Governments may, as Archard points out, harm children by
conscripting them into military service or by denying them food,
shelter and health care, but does this necessarily make them evil? Evil
in the eyes of their enemies perhaps, but not in the eyes of their
friends. It is easy to talk of evil leaders in ways that attribute all the
ills perpetrated by a country or government to a particular individual
or to particular individuals, but is it really possible to refer to
ministries or courts or other institutions as evil or abusive? Clearly
Archard believes that it is, while an autopoietic systems analysis would
see the operation of such organizations as morally neutral and immune
from moral judgements, except in so far as they were succeeding or
failing to perform their functions in the way that the system itself had
laid down for their effective operation (see King, Chapter 1, pp. 6–9).

Corruption, nepotism, discrimination, inequality are all terms that may be validly directed against a social system's operation, but this does not make the system itself bad in its own terms, unless these failings adversely affect the system's operations. The 'problems' come not from within, but from moral judgements made outside the system. For example, a system within an 'evil' regime, such as that for the deportation and extermination of Jews in Nazi Germany, may run extremely efficiently. Here the value judgements of evil, repulsive and abusive are applied to the system and by those outside the system who believe that they have the moral authority to make such judgements. Others are entitled to disagree with them by arguing, for example, for a different version of morality or for a different source of moral authority.

To some extent Archard tackles these difficulties when he considers cultural variations where the beliefs and values of one culture are brought to bear in passing moral judgements on the values and practices of another. As he rightly points out, 'The belief that there is a single standard of morally acceptable behaviour towards children, and that this standard is to be found operating in our own society, may rest upon ethnocentric assumptions of cultural superiority.' Yet actively to avoid making any moral judgements where standards for the treatment of children are markedly lower than our own runs the risk of moral relativism. Quite how one avoids falling into one or other of these two traps is not clear.

One possible escape from this dilemma is to let science decide once and for all what is good and bad for children, what constitutes abuse and what does not, and so avoid accusations of moral relativism. According to Ilan Katz (Chapter 6), the most obvious reason why 'male circumcision can be seen as morally wrong…is that circumcision involves physically injuring the child' and so 'transgresses…the right of children to physical integrity'. To follow this line of reasoning is to conclude that 'all physical harm to children is unacceptable, unless it is done for medical reasons'. This, as Katz recognizes, is a difficult argument to sustain when faced with cultural traditions, such as facial scarring, neck elongation or circumcision which may be seen, through the eyes of an external observer, to be causing injury to the child, but which, from within the culture, are perceived as essential to the child's identity and to traditional values. The same medically founded criterion of harm has also been deployed against smacking children, but it need not confine itself to physical harm. It is frequently applied to emotional or psychological injury to children, the only difference being that evidence of injury in such cases may be more controversial and difficult to establish. Yet few would argue that definitions of harms to children should be confined to those that medical science recognizes as injurious, but may include a range of other harms, such as damage to a child's identity, innocence, integrity, self-confidence, etc. Once it is established that moral harm is not necessarily equivalent to physical or psychological injuries, it is no longer possible to appoint science as the judge of moral values. Of course, the tendency today is for every aspect of children's lives to be reconstituted as amenable to scientific investigation and pronouncement, but wherever these pronouncements go beyond descriptions of physical phenomena and enter the normative debate about what is good or bad for children (and not just for children's bodies) they rely on moral assumptions. And so we are forced to return to moral philosophers, such as David Archard in this book, to question these assumptions.

The second problem faced by scientific attempts to resolve moral issues is, as Katz recognizes, that science exists within a particular culture, and those who apply scientific knowledge in their work as professionals charged with protecting children from abuse 'must work within the system of thought, *and of morality*, which is characteristic of Western liberal professionalism' (emphasis added). Other cultures do not appoint science to the exalted position of supreme judge. Moreover, they also sustain very different versions of morality from the 'Western, liberal'. These versions of morality may provide very different notions of what is good or bad for children than the child welfare professionals. The answer to the question at the end of Ilan Katz's chapter, 'Could it be possible that some behaviours can be abusive but also morally defensible?', has to be 'no'. To define behaviour as abusive is itself a moral judgement, so that abusive behaviour will necessarily be morally indefensible. On the other hand, those moral systems which treat as acceptable behaviour such as male or female circumcision will, also by definition, see them as morally defensible. We are forced to return to the question of 'whose morality?'

The morality of successful parenting

Marinos Diamantides in Chapter 7 somewhat unfashionably expresses his disappointment at the decline of paternalism in modern Western history. While private individuals, including parents, may respond to those who are unable to cater for their own needs in a paternalistic way, the modern democratic state finds it difficult to do so. For the state to attempt such paternalism risks revealing the fact that individual needs cannot be met by social reciprocity, '"one-way" actions of paternalistic generosity'. To mobilize public resources for the sake of individual needs risks undermining the very paternalistic 'generosity' which has answered such needs, for example, as those associated with bringing up children or looking after sick parents.

On the other hand, the unpopularity of paternalism today, according to Diamantides, also results from the belief, in the absence of any objective reality, that to detect needs in others is a projection of the 'subjective preferences' and values of the actor and may thus be seen as an expression of the paternalists' self-interest in constructing others in their own image. The modern state, therefore, has to temper any impulse to be kind with the 'principles of individual autonomy, consent and self-determination'. The result is that the 'right' of each individual to have their person and body protected from 'intrusion' is seen as overriding the 'paternalistic' desires of parents, lovers and carers. Similarly, paternalistic behaviour is permissible only if it can be seen to further the other person's autonomy and cannot be justified on the grounds of mere welfare (as interpreted by the paternalist). For parents to treat children as if they were simply a duplication of their (adult) self and as such endowed with a capacity to exercise autonomy is equally open to criticism, for not recognizing the 'otherness' of the child. In both these anti-paternalist instances the child does not represent that unique being that arouses compassion and anxiety in its parents on account of its very uniqueness. Rather, in the case of a welfare or needs approach, the projection onto the child of the special needs of minors denies the child's existence as an other whose company the parents may enjoy; in the case of rights attribution, liberal parents do not assert their concern for the circumstances of their 'immature child' and so end up by *'being* their children'. In both cases, according to Diamantides, there is a denial of parental responsibility, which makes for unsuccessful parenting.

Yet for Diamantides these two agendas need not be treated as if they were mutually exclusive. He draws on the concept of 'fecundity' as expounded by the moral philosopher, Emmanuel Levinas (Levinas, 1969). For Levinas, the love of parents for their child (or for any human being who cares for another) is able to break free from the past and present. In expressing their parenthood, parents transcend themselves and yet retain their identity. The abstract idea of 'child' and 'adult' enables the parent to open themselves to *the idea of infinity*, liberated from the continuity of past and present. In relating to the child 'the adult comes to transcend the realm of the possible' and to respond to a future not yet in existence, but which matters now. By applying this notion of fecundity it is possible to resolve the deadlock between caring for the child's immediate welfare and promoting the child's absolute autonomy. The conflict between them ends when we stop seeing them as opposites or, alternatively, when we see them separately with reference to a vision of the future where justice coincides with care.

Applying these ideas, Diamantides refuses to join most legal commentators on children's rights in their celebration of the landmark English case of *Gillick v West Norfolk and Wisbech Area Health Authority*. He does not share with them their vision of the momentous significance of the House of Lords' radical departure from a past refusal of the law to recognize the possibility of children's autonomy and its entry into a new era of children's rights. On the contrary, he sees the judgement as a missed opportunity. Rather than construing children as autonomous and capable of defying their parents in deciding issues of medical treatment, the judges symbolically separated the Gillick children from their parents and placed them under their patronage. They simply substituted their evaluation of what the child needed for that of the parents, and wrapped up their decision in the rhetoric of rights. The decision was one in which 'priority was given to the need of modern children to have direct access to medical advice on contraceptives over any conflicting needs that biological parents invoke'. Diamantides sees this as *bad* parental talk of the 'magisterial' type. It did not take the form of a loving intervention, an assumption of responsibility by the judges and an apology for their inevitable 'subjectivism'. Rather, it was an impersonal proclamation of the law with regard to the child.

The lawfulness of injustice

Diamantides' critique of the Gillick decision poses once again the crucial question as to whether social systems such as law are capable of moral judgements. He clearly believes that they are and sees no difficulties in people who are acting in their capacity as teachers or judges adopting the same moral approach to minors as parents. Alison Diduck, on the other hand, is not so optimistic. At the end of her contribution (Chapter 8) she recognizes, in her admission that she has no plan or blueprint as to the process for bridging the gap between liberal law and morality, that attempts to bring into law a notion of justice that resides outside the legal system is fraught with difficulties.

She is a critic of the legal system's tendency in its communications to construct one-dimensional people who are either dependent or independent, who are either competent individuals or subjects in need of protection. She complains of the law's failure to operate a version of

justice which integrates all the attributes of human beings, preordained by the categories 'child' and 'adult', instead of focusing only on
those which conform with a single image of the person with which it is
dealing. She sees some hope for change, however, in the present crisis
over the meaning of childhood, which, she claims, has had the effect of
collapsing, or at least, blurring the distinction between adults and children. Once this distinction can no longer be relied upon for the
production of reductionist, generalized and universalized legal categories that enable law to reach simplistic conclusions as to what is and
what is not good for children, the legal system may be obliged to recast
its normative conception of what justice means for children. Once freed
from the need to think in terms of boundaries between adults and children, dependence and independence, etc., law, she hopes, will be able
'to take account of an individual's multiplicity of qualities as both
"legal" and "moral" subject'. The effects of this crisis of childhood,
brought about by the phenomenon of adult-like children, is likely to
alter law's concepts of justice for children and adults alike. It will
enable law to see people as they really are, as connected to others in
complex ways and as situated in their own particular environment.

Her position is one of 'a moralist', one who views law from the
outside, from a vantage point which enables her to see the inadequacies
and inequities of generalized legal constructs when compared with the
nuanced nature of 'real people's' existence. The misfit between law's
conception of child welfare and what is good or bad, just or unjust for
individual children can be seen in legal decisions, such as those
mandating 'the wholesale removal of aboriginal children from their
families in both Canada and Australia and their placement with
"white" families'. Yet this example also highlights the difficulties with
her critical stance, for at the time that these legal decisions were taken,
they appeared to be morally sound. Only in retrospect have they been
shown to be bad, that is contrary to the interests of the child. This may
be because time has revealed the suffering of these children and the
emotional damage inflicted on them, or because moral values have
changed and today the close relationship between birth parents and
their children is seen as more valuable than in the past. These two
reasons may, of course, be causally interconnected, with psychological
evidence feeding moral values and moral values providing an impetus
for psychological research. Whatever the relation between them, it
would not have been possible for the courts at the time of these decisions to know that what appeared at the time to conform to moral as
well as legal notions of justice would turn out at some future date to
have been legal but immoral. Law does not know what it cannot see.

Diduck's critique then forces us, as well as the legal system, to confront the fraught question of 'whose morality?' If there were people around in Australia and Canada at the time who were opposed to the removal of aboriginal children, should the courts have heeded their objections? What if these objections were never raised in court, so that the judges were presented with a simple choice between an inadequate or dysfunctional aboriginal family and a perfect white family? Perhaps the generalized and universalized categories that Alison Diduck complains of serve as empty vessels which may be filled with whatever moral values or whatever versions of child welfare happen to be prevalent at the time. In this way law itself may remain neutral or amoral, while making itself available for different moral accounts at different times and in different places. If law is to embrace 'the real child' and answer its 'real needs', then somewhere outside the legal system there has to exist some authoritative way of identifying what is 'real'. Otherwise we cannot go beyond moral rhetoric, enticing as this moral rhetoric may appear. The risk that Alison Diduck and, to some extent, Andrew Cooper (Chapter 10) run in their demand for law to be formulated in ways which relate to children and adults as subjects in all their complexity and completeness is that the version of 'reality' (and of morality) that law adopts may not meet with their approval.

The morality of therapy

Judith Trowell and Gillian Miles (Chapter 9) share with other contributors a quest to unravel the complexities that occur when attempts are made to apply moral principles to institutionalized practices for the promotion of children's welfare, which have been built on different bodies of knowledge and understanding than morality. Difficulties arise, for example, between moral imperatives and psychoanalytic practices when analytical psychotherapists become involved in protecting children against abuse by parents. The need for psychoanalysts to withhold judgement and 'stay within the realm of uncertainty' conflicts directly with demands for definitive statements of cause and effect, and the unambiguous attributions of responsibility that society demands from its experts. By immersing themselves too deeply in the internal world of their patients, psychotherapists may fail to recognize that they are part of society and that their therapeutic communications are not immune from being evaluated as morally right or morally wrong (as feminist critiques of psychoanalysis have made only too clear) or being reproduced as moral judgements on others.

This relationship between morality and therapy is also taken up by

Andrew Cooper in Chapter 10. Like Marinos Diamantides in his support of 'fecundity', he wants decision-makers who confront issues of children's welfare to respond to the child in a way which recognizes the child's total being, including the social and relational context in which the child exists. Like Alison Diduck, he voices his concerns over the conventional version of justice which is at present dispensed by the courts in Britain, and which influences much of the thinking and practice of welfare agencies in relation to child abuse. It is a form of justice which, he claims, fails to tackle the complexity of interpersonal relationships or to enter the minds of the children that it is supposed to serve. Complexity, as identified, for example, by the social theorists, Michael Walzer and John Gray, can find no expression within the adversarial nature of the courtroom contest. Likewise, the inner self of the child cannot be recognized by a legal system which cannot cope with multiple truth and inherent uncertainty. Cooper argues for courts which are more 'therapeutic in their approach to human predicaments in which the connections between the intra-psychic, interpersonal and social dimensions are central'. He wants to see a specialist system of law which is tailored to the particular needs of child welfare, which is able to deal with interpersonal issues and to 'come into direct relationship with those who have been exposed to the traumatic and irrational'.

Faced with the problems of translating principles of interpersonal relations into institutional (or social system) settings which were discussed in Chapter 1, it is difficult to conceptualize a legal system which is capable of adopting Andrew Cooper's particular moral agenda. He points to the legal and child protection systems of continental Europe as in some ways fulfilling his demands for a specialized justice, but even in these countries, this is made possible only by the withdrawal of law from making judgements about the relationship between parents and children, preferring to leave such matters to child welfare expertise. It is the medico-therapeutic communications of the experts which become accepted as authoritative on what is good/bad parenting and what is good/bad for children. The essential nature of law's role in these countries is not different from its role in the United Kingdom. It is rather that decisions concerning the welfare of children are not considered to be legal issues (or are less often considered to be legal issues), and are left to other systems where the coding of sick/healthy, normal/pathological creates the expectation of different certainties from those of the legal system. A child or family is in need of treatment for 'their problems' or is not in need of treatment, is being treated or is not being treated, has responded to treatment or has not responded. For those concerned with the emotional development of the child or the relationship between that child and its family, this may well be a better way of protecting children than insisting that the courts reach a decision on whether the parent is or is not 'a child abuser', but it is not necessarily more moral. Only by conflating morality (or justice) with the mental health of children is it possible to see this contest between law and therapy in moral terms. Yet it is perhaps not surprising that child therapists should oppose legal justice when confronted with a legal system that is capable of, for example, insisting that the more serious the allegations of abuse the stronger the burden of proof and so making it all the less likely that the abuse will be officially recognized.[2]

Child sexuality and morality

The transience and instability of moral discourses concerning children is an issue which Wendy and Rex Stainton Rogers discuss in their chapter on children's sexuality (Chapter 11). They criticize the current moral 'censorship of childhood sexuality' which 'takes the form of simply denying it and refusing to accept that there can be any form of sex that is "good" for children', because of the 'terrible harm that is wrought by any kind of sexual experience in childhood'. Their critique is in part directed against the paradoxical state of the law which recognizes the capacity of children for sexual behaviour with one breath and tries to protect them against any sexual experience with the next but, more fundamentally, it is an attack on a certain kind of hypocrisy which claims the knowledge to deny children any freedom to enjoy sex, while at the same time endorsing the widespread exploitation of children by adults as sexual objects in advertising and fashion modelling. It is a moral critique of moralizers who, through the rhetorical appeal of their rigid moral agendas, have succeeded both in constructing children as objects in need of protection from any kind of sexual experience and in silencing anyone who is unwise enough to challenge this account.

The Stainton Rogers draw on Michel Foucault's analysis of sexuality as an 'especially dense transfer point for relations of power' (Foucault, 1990, pp. 104–5). Like Foucault, they approach morality from a polit-ical perspective and from this vantage point are able to identify the power strategies that are brought into play around sexual issues. Where children are concerned, the issue of consent, they argue, has become an important locus for such power games. While children are increasingly seen as competent to participate in decision-making about matters which affect them, it is still assumed that they are incapable of consenting to sex. Why should this be? One answer lies in the way in which a moralizing discourse concerning sex and children has been used politically by some feminist writers in their attack on male sexual exploitation of children as an example of patriarchy. Another answer may be found in the child welfare professions, where protecting children against sexual abuse has become a major growth industry creating a vested interest in the continuing management of child sexual abuse as a social problem and so in denying children any autonomy in decisions concerning sex. The Stainton Rogers see the combination of these two discourses as hegemonic and authoritarian and, therefore, to be resisted. In doing so they invoke a higher morality than that of the moralizers, a moral agenda which recognizes child sexuality and allows the possibility that it might be expressed in ways which are not always harmful to children.

Religion and morality

Stephen Frosh, in Chapter 12, tackles moral authoritarianism of a different kind, that which he identifies as being dispensed by religious fundamentalism. Whereas morality, as we have seen, is a way of communicating about people in terms of their goodness or badness, religion is able to reproduce such judgements as having been made by some superior being or force residing outside society. Moral principles are transformed into laws which are of divine origin. For fundamentalists, these laws must be obeyed without question, even if they conflict with the morality of the external, secular world. To disobey is not only wrong, it also strikes at the heart of religious identity. It lays the deviant open to opprobrium and even to expulsion from the religious community. For those, like Frosh, who approach morality from a liberal perspective, which champions freedom of choice for the individual, religious fundamentalism of the kind that finds expression in the evangelism of the American New Christian Right, in Islamic terrorism or in the murders committed in Israel by members of right-wing Jewish sects is frightening and dangerous, above all because it is willing 'to snuff out dissent'. But Frosh also recognizes its seductive appeal at a time in history when, if postmodernists are correct, life has become fragmented and few certainties exist for people to cling on to.

For religious fundamentalists, even more than for the rest of society, children represent an investment in the future. For them the very survival of the community depends upon the instillation of their traditional values in each new generation. For them, 'the best interests of the child' must give way to 'the best interests of the community'. Duty takes precedence over personal fulfilment: 'preservation of the community and its traditional values is of paramount concern in fundamentalist cultures – passing down the truth to the next generation'. Children belong to the community and not to themselves. Moral responsibility towards children does not consist of educating a child in such a way that he or she will eventually be free 'to choose between the array of careers and lifestyles on offer in the West'. On the contrary, it is to educate the child in such a way that this freedom is not recognized, or where it is recognized, that it is rejected. It is personal freedom, the cult of the individual, which, according to the fundamentalist perspective, leads to rootlessness, immorality, materialism and self-destruction among young people. Fundamentalism, therefore, confronts liberal moralists with a moral agenda for children which flies in the face of their most treasured principles. It undermines any attempts by communitarians or pluralists to erect or resurrect the concept of a consensual or universal morality, a moral code to which everyone is willing to subscribe. Indeed, Frosh in his chapter criticizes multiculturalism for its endorsement of extremist views in its naïve attempt to forge a society where all cultures are given equal tolerance and respect.

Stephen Frosh seems to suggest in his concluding remarks that it is possible to defeat fundamentalism on moral as well as political grounds. While the activities of fundamentalists may well be restrained politically by the simple device of starving them of power, and, for that matter, legally, by declaring their most extreme activities to be unlawful, it is difficult to see how morality could be deployed against them except by making dubious claims of higher authority. Who is to judge the rival claims that right (and not might) is on their side? Science may be the answer, as Ilan Katz illustrates in his chapter on male circumcision (Chapter 6). If it can be shown scientifically that religious practices are medically (whether physically or psychologically) bad for children, then, in a society which accepts scientific truth as 'the truth', there may be a possibility of resolving conflicts between rival moral claims. Yet, once again, there is no guarantee that this will occur. A more likely scenario may be the one that Katz identifies: that of two or more moral systems existing side by side with no possibility of the one communicating directly with the other and no way of determining definitively which one is right.

Moral judgements in school

Daniel Monk poses a different question, again concerning science and morality, but this time in the sphere of education. When (if at all) should moral judgements be constrained or withheld altogether in the interests of a child's welfare. This is a question which is continually being raised in relation to children who commit crimes, where it takes the form of a debate between punishment and welfare. Present trends are in favour of punishment in part as a political solution to reassure the electorate that tough measures are being taken against juvenile criminals, but also, at a psychological level, to encourage children to take responsibility for their actions. Increasingly the same issues are having to be faced in the field of education, where a choice has to be made as to whether moral/legal or welfare/therapeutic measures are called for. The solution that has been adopted by the Department for Education in England is to draw a line between children having special needs and children who are so disruptive that they should be excluded from school. While moral judgements are withheld for the first category, with the children being treated as having problems not of their own making which are in need of remedial action, those who are labelled as 'disruptive' are subjected to legalistic disciplinary procedures – the exclusion proceedings – which concentrate on the conduct of the pupil and subject that conduct to moral judgements. For the first group, it is the child's disability that gives rise to a need; for the second, it is the child's refusal to obey the rules and behave as an ideal pupil that warrants action to protect the interests of other children at the school: 'the former focuses on what the child has done and can be blamed for, while the latter focuses on what a child appears unable to do'.

Children's 'needs' in education, according to Monk, 'can be identified clearly in the scientific discipline of developmental psychology', but when 'special needs' enters the educational arena (as it does in the Education Act 1966) it does so as a term with a very specific meaning: 'it is not learning per se that is crucial in the diagnosis of a special educational need, but rather the ability to learn particular knowledge in a particular way'. Similarly, the term, 'disability', once politically sanctioned, may be used for the discovery, promotion and extension of a plethora of clinical disorders, such as dyslexia and attention deficit disorder. The diagnosis of such a disorder in a child immediately takes the matter outside the sphere of morality into that of science, so removing any personal responsibility for behaviour. This is of particular interest in relation to attention deficit disorder, since behaviour which falls under this category may also fall within the category of disruptive behaviour warranting school exclusion which has clear moral implications. It is by no means clear what the criteria are by which children fall on one side of this moral divide or the other. Just as in the juvenile justice system children may be somewhat arbitrarily divided into depraved and deprived, into those deserving punishment and those needing treatment, so in education politically constructed categories are used to locate the ill-defined and non-specific behaviour of some children within a morally charged discourse and of other children within a scientific/therapeutic system which appears morally neutral.

Notes

1 Chris Jenks' recent book, *Childhood* (1996), gives a social constructionist account of these different images of children.
2 Re H and R, [1996] 1FLR 80.

3 Moral campaigns for children's welfare in the nineteenth century

Christine Piper

As the clouds of pessimism gathered in the late 1980s and 1990s, it was increasingly accepted that there was an historical legacy that needed to be better understood.

(Cox, 1996, p. 4)[1]

Introduction

The construction of child abuse and, in particular, child sexual abuse, as a major social problem in the last quarter of the twentieth century has led to renewed interest in historical material about child abuse and neglect. In particular, it has stimulated a re-examination of what have been referred to as 'moral campaigns' against child cruelty which occurred in the nineteenth century. The implication of that title is that what was happening to children was morally wrong – an evil to be eradicated. Several generations of school children have therefore learnt about children climbing chimneys, going down mines, working in factories and living on the streets, and of the efforts of people such as Lord Shaftesbury, Mary Carpenter and Dr Barnardo to give them homes and improve their conditions of work, or to remove them from employment or imprisonment. A quotation from a children's book of the 1950s gives the flavour of this approach:

Many of the changes in our lives have been made not by rulers or statesmen but by reformers – men and women who realised that something was seriously wrong and who strove to set it right....

In the early factories the workers were badly treated. Men, women and even young children were forced to toil for many hours each day in dreadful conditions. Two great reformers led the way to overcoming these evils. Lord Shaftesbury got laws passed limiting the hours and regulating the conditions of work: Robert

Owen ran his factory on humane lines, and encouraged cooperative enterprise rather than competition.

(*Odhams Encyclopaedia for Children, c.* 1954, p. 204)

Study of those campaigns has, therefore, until relatively recently, been in a liberal historical tradition which, beginning with the historians of the Enlightenment, had focused on cause and consequence.[2] Historians with that approach looked for signs of progress, analysed who was responsible for achieving the reforms and assumed that, as knowledge accumulated within the historical period under review, there would be further progress towards a possible utopia where all evils were overcome. The assimilation of Marxist and sociological approaches to historical research led only to a change of emphasis from individual agents to those economic conditions which facilitated or provoked change and those class- and gender-based interests through which change occurred.[3] Questions of how and why certain actions were labelled evil and why there was a focus on a particular evil at any point in time continued to be begged. The influence on historical research of postmodernism – with its undermining of optimism and the role of 'grand theory' – was therefore immense.[4]

In particular, analysis of time- and place-specific discourses which constrain and mould patterns of thought (as exemplified by the work of Foucault)[5] and the work of sociologists of deviance (who focused on responses to 'nonconforming' behaviour as defining that behaviour) have allowed of very different interpretations of the nature of moral campaigns against child cruelty in the nineteenth century. Research such as that of Becker (1963) and Gusfield (1963)[6] introduced a focus on the processes by which evil and morality themselves were constructed: what is right or wrong at any point in time could no longer be taken for granted. The nature of the analytical exercise then becomes that of constructing contemporary meanings for the terms 'moral crusades' and 'moral entrepreneurs' and defining the nature and influence of the 'moral' element as it relates to the focus for reform. As a result, my aim is not to determine whether humanitarian reformers and religious zeal *or* economic change determined the nature, timing and outcome of the 'crusades' in relation to the welfare of children. This chapter is a more modest exercise. Its aim is to find out what (and why) particular moral truths were being constructed and drawn upon to influence outcomes in relevant decades.

There is now historical material available to answer this question: the genesis of, and moral frameworks for, both institutionalized philanthropic activity and legislation addressing the welfare of children in the Victorian and Edwardian periods have been analysed from several standpoints. Current interest in the origins of concern about child abuse has generated further documentary research on individuals and societies campaigning against child cruelty at the end of the nineteenth century. Theoretical interest in forms of social control and regulation has led to analysis (using notions of normalization and tutelage) of the role of 'lady visitors' and, later, health visitors, school medical inspections and delinquency prevention projects, for example. This particular focus has also led to a concentration (e.g. in the work of Eekelaar and Dingwall[7]) on the effect of such intervention on the distinction between the public and the private. Writers such as Becker (1963) and Platt (1969) have researched responses to juvenile deviance to analyse class-based moralities and struggles to confirm status. More recently, material from these periods has been plundered, particularly by those writing under the aegis of the Institute of Economic Affairs, to explain the nature of Victorian values and virtues, or the advantages of charitable rather than state organization of 'welfare' (e.g. Himmelfarb, 1995 and Whelan, 1996). In addition, work on concepts of childhood (Stainton Rogers and Stainton Rogers, 1992; Cunningham, 1995; Cox, 1996) and on children's rights (Freeman, 1983; Archard, 1993) offer new perspectives on the wealth of material in standard sociological histories of childhood, notably Pinchbeck and Hewitt (1969, 1973).

What this chapter aims to do is to use the insights provided by these different approaches to analyse in more detail the nature of the moral agendas being pursued, and to identify more clearly different historical perceptions of how children were being 'wronged': what did reformers construct as 'seriously wrong' and who were the 'enemies' of children that the reformers were fighting? This chapter, therefore, seeks to disaggregate the perceived consensual Victorian moral agenda for the improvement of the welfare of children and to show how far and in what ways the 'wrongs' to be put right related to perceived moral needs of the reformers and society as well as identified wrongs done to children.

The visible Victorian child

It would be quite misleading to suggest that the child was ignored and invisible before the nineteenth century. However, the development of ideas of innocence and malleability in connection with children replacing, at least to an extent, a concept of original sin, together with a much clearer sense of the separation of childhood and adulthood, led to a greater focus on the role of childhood and to the treatment of children.[8] In that sense, as Behlmer points out, 'the mid-Victorian generation gave unprecedented attention to children and the problems facing them' (Behlmer, 1982, p. 3). The image of the child which resulted was a sentimental image of a child who was also frequently portrayed as a vulnerable victim. Behlmer draws attention particularly to the work of Charles Dickens for images of children as 'reservoirs of sensitivity' and to the speeches of Lord Shaftesbury for examples of what he refers to as the 'politics of pathos' (*ibid.*). The popular pictures of children – even those of children who had not been neglected – are images of children who are especially sensitive and often physically weak. As Hendrick (1994) argues, by the last quarter of the nineteenth century the focus of philanthropic and state attention was on the body (as opposed to the mind) of the child, but the image of the child which had by then become authoritative was one which evoked the physical fragility of the child – the reverse of the developing image of the 'muscular Christian' adult male.

These weak, sensitive, vulnerable children have no 'voice' of their own, however. Elizabeth Barrett Browning's 'The Cry of the Children' (1843),[9] Andrew Mearn's 'The Bitter Cry of Outcast London' (1883) and John Spargo's 'The Bitter Cry of the Children' ([1906] 1969)[10] all evoke an image of those who silently 'cry'; who are victims because they have no ability or power to articulate 'aloud' their needs.[11] The powerlessness of the child is what, paradoxically, gives the image such power. As Sadler expressed it, when urging support for the Ten Hours Bill 1832, 'I wish I could bring a group of these little ones to [the] bar [of the House of Commons] – I am sure their silent appearance would plead more forcibly in their behalf than the loudest eloquence.'[12]

Childhood had not only become accepted as a separate and different first stage of life but the concern, as Cunningham points out, became one which focused on 'children without a childhood'.[13] Before the 1880s the powerful images of the victim/child were those of children who were both most visibly and most publicly being denied a childhood – children who were 'outside' the family because they were working in factories and mines. The existence of large numbers of such children was a relatively new development[14] resulting from industrialization. Social and economic developments which are both new and visible provoke fear: a notable example occurred in Tudor times. The existence of a new class of wandering landless labourers in the sixteenth century caused widespread panic reflected in the first two lines of a nursery rhyme – 'Hark, hark, the dogs do bark, / The beggars are coming to town' – and became a major influence on the nature of

Poor Law legislation. By the early nineteenth century, industrialization was similarly being feared as a force which threatened to destroy rural life and family-, or quasi-family-, centred life, which people knew and understood.[15] As 'moral panic' theorists have made clear,[16] where such social fear of changing conditions exists there is receptive ground for those who argue for action against a perceived resulting evil. Those campaigning in the early and middle part of the nineteenth century to better the lives of children therefore tackled what was the most easily seen evil – that produced by the workplace, particularly the new workplaces[17] which put children beyond the reach of protection by their parents. Not only that, the evil was two-headed: the potential or actual harm to children was both physical and moral. The new workplaces were seen as the source of deprivation and depravity.

And so legislation to protect children first dealt with apprentices, servant girls, chimney sweeps and then factory owners.[18] Nor did agitation for, or implementation of, such employment legislation cease when the main focus of concern later became that of cruelty to children in the home. Concern with the protection of children from the cruelties inflicted by capitalism continued throughout the century: in the twenty years after the inaugural meeting of the Liverpool Society for the Prevention of Cruelty to Children, in 1883, were passed the Coal Mines and Stratified Ironstone Mines Amendment Act 1887, the Factory and Workshop Amending Acts of 1891 and 1901, the Shop Hours Act 1892, the Mines (Prohibition of Child Labour Underground) Act 1900 and the Employment (Children) Act 1903.

The same concern was apparent in other jurisdictions facing similar stages of industrialization. For example, the introduction to 'The Bitter Cry of the Children' (Spargo, [1906] 1969) pointed out that the aim of the book's author – a Cornishman who had emigrated to the USA – was 'to make us see that "this great nation in its commercial madness devours its babes"'. This image of 'babes' is invoked throughout his book, though the author is referring to the 1.7 million children and young people under sixteen who were gainfully employed according to the 1900 census in the United States of America, rather than to 'babies' as the late twentieth century would use the term. Again the image is of a child so physically weak and dependent that 'babe' is an appropriate image.

This idea of physical dependency, in conjunction with the 'urban disenchantment' which Platt discusses in relation to influences on nineteenth-century images of North American children (Platt, 1969, pp. 36–43), fed also into ideas of the inherent evil of the very streets which children outside the family experience.[19] What emerged was the idea that children should not be publicly visible: that it is wrong to allow a child to act as an adult, either by working in particular places or by being 'independent' on the streets – an idea which is still powerful in relation to campaigns to protect 'street children' in developing countries.[20]

That the protection of children from the evils of employment was a priority for reformers, and subsequently for the state, from the end of the eighteenth century is, therefore, relatively understandable. The more difficult questions are why intervention in the family to protect children occurred as late as it did and why it occurred to protect delinquent children earlier than abused children. Here there is a problem, for my purposes, with some of the literature. The aim, for example, of the analysis by Dingwall *et al.* (1984) of the historical origins of legislation relating to child care and protection is to specify which motives (of campaigners and/or the government) explain satisfactorily the introduction, passage and implementation of legislation. They therefore draw particularly, as does Hendrick (1994), on the apparently dichotomous images of the child as victim or threat, and focus on the importance of the moral socialization of children in a liberal state.

The fear of inadequate socialization of children was undoubtedly an impetus for reform throughout the nineteenth century: the comments of factory and child welfare reformers make that clear.

> The saving of the industrial child reflects a moral concern: the presence of women and children in industry was repeatedly linked to *their* depravity. The picture of vice and indecency in factories and mines was drawn as much to point to the dangers of a demoralised working class...as to protest on behalf of child victims.
>
> (Cannan, 1992, p. 53)

The motivations of politicians would of necessity include concern for the future needs of the state: 'Children were thought to be unformed enough to be saveable. They represented the future' (Cunningham, 1995, p. 135). But as Gordon points out in her study of the Massachusetts' Society for the Prevention of Cruelty to Children,

> The fit between child-saving and other social anxieties was an historical fact, not a causal explanation. Their concern about children was not merely a mask for intervention whose 'real' purposes were other.... However, their own values and anxieties made that cruelty more visible and disturbing than it had once been.
>
> (Gordon, 1988, p. 30)

This suggests that it may be both unhelpful and impossible to try and disentangle motivations to decide whether the concern was for the unhappy child per se or for the future demoralized citizen. Instead, my focus will be on isolating those particular anxieties that allowed for shifts in the Victorian moral framework held by those classes whose support in the passage and implementation of legislation was crucial. The rest of this chapter will look more closely at the campaigns responding to child criminality (culminating in the 1857 Industrial Schools Act) and to cruelty to infants and children (culminating in the Infant Life Preservation Act 1872 and the 'anti-cruelty' Act of 1889) to see how significant shifts occurred in the 1850s and 1880s. Why did a concern for the effective moral socialization of children lead to different successful campaigns at different times? Dingwall *et al.* said of the industrial schools movement: 'For reasons which are not altogether clear...there was no major legislation until the middle of the century' (1984, p. 215). To shed light on those reasons it is helpful to start with a look at why legislation to protect children from cruelty within their families did not reach the statute book until the end of the 1880s.

The lesser of two evils?

The assumption has been made that parental abuse was at this time simply constructed as excessive discipline[21] and was therefore not considered evil. Recent research would suggest that this is not true: there was acknowledgement that domestic abuse occurred by the mid-nineteenth century and violence in the family was no longer being constructed socially as normal. Pollock's analysis of newspaper accounts of prosecutions of parents for cruelty suggests they were not uncommon in the period 1784 to 1860, and she quotes magisterial comment which explicitly rebuts the idea that 'the father had a right to do as he pleased' (Pollock, 1983, pp. 62–4).[22] It was therefore something to be denounced and one example of such denunciation was the Act for Better Prevention of Aggravated Assaults 1853 though, as Behlmer points out, it was used more to protect women: research shows little evidence of prosecution of offenders under this Act in regard to assaults on children.

The evil of cruelty to children within the family was apparent before the 1880s. Within the context of moral imperatives for action, therefore, the answer appears simple – interfering with parents' rights was at that time constructed as a greater evil than that of child abuse. What is often quoted in support of this conclusion is the reply of Lord

Shaftesbury in 1871 to a letter asking for his support for legislation to protect children from parental cruelty, in which he wrote

> the evils you state are enormous and indisputable, but they are of so private, internal and domestic a character as to be beyond the reach of legislation, and the subject, indeed, would not, I think, be entertained by either House of Parliament.[23]

The same attitude is apparent in those philanthropists responding to family poverty. For example, the 1889 Annual Report of the Charity Organisation Society said 'everything should be done to help distress in such a way that it does not become a matter rather of public than of private concern' and C.S. Loch, who was appointed honorary secretary of the COS in 1875, wrote, 'not to give arms but to keep alive the saving health of the family becomes its problem'.[24]

Those who, in support of the moral necessity of family autonomy, suggested the state had never interfered in the family were of course wrong, as Pinchbeck and Hewitt point out when quoting Cooke Taylor's comment of 1874:'That unit, the family, is the unit upon which a constitutional Government has been raised which is the admiration and envy of mankind. Hitherto, whatever the laws have touched, they have not invaded this sacred precinct...' (Pinchbeck and Hewitt, 1973, p. 359).

The state had intervened to restrict or remove the rights of the parents and guardians of both rich and poor children via the wardship powers of the courts and the duties of the Poor Law Authorities. Restrictions on the parental rights of the economically dependent clearly did not 'count'.[25] Parental cruelty to children was therefore simply not wicked enough to balance out the evils of interference with parental control and, particularly, of interference with the rights of a wage-earning father.

On one level this appears quite incomprehensible to the late twentieth-century mind because religion no longer has the authority which it had for the Victorians. The prevalent Victorian Christian religious truth was that the father is the 'natural' head of the family, and that he requires the moral, religious and actual authority of that position to ensure the family is run as a unit which transmits the moral values of society. This divinely ordered system would achieve the welfare of the greatest number of children and families. Without unfettered power and responsibility to organize and discipline for the good of the family, the father could not fulfil that role properly: it was therefore seen as too dangerous to risk intervening in families to investigate abuse of the parental power.

The Victorian moral crusaders were part of a society that took this particular system of morality for granted. When these crusaders spoke of the need to change people's ideas in order to protect the child, they spoke within a system of morality that was taken as unchallengeable. It would therefore be wrong to assume that, until the 1880s, those campaigning to eradicate the evils of child abuse were frustrated by a system of morality to which they did not subscribe.[26] They upheld the need for an autonomous family unit as essential to the moral health of the nation.

That the crusaders so constrained themselves is clear from the following speech in the House of Commons by Lord Ashley[27] (later Lord Shaftesbury) in 1844. He discussed child labour before moving on to the question of female labour, referring to the report of the Medical Officer of Stockport which stated that 'it has been the practice in mills, gradually to dispense with the labour of males'. He then made the following point which I will extract at some length:

> But listen to another fact and one deserving of serious attention; that the females not only perform the labour but occupy the places of men; they are forming various clubs and associations, and gradually acquiring all those privileges which are held to be the proper portion of the male sex....Here is a dialogue which occurred in one of these clubs, from an eyewitness:- 'A man came into one of these clubrooms, with a child in his arms; "Come lass," said he addressing one of the single women, "come home for I cannot keep this bairn quiet, and the other one I have left crying at home": "I won't go home, idle devil", she replied, "I have thee to keep and the bairns too, and if I can't get a pint of ale quietly, it is tiresome...I won't go home yet"'. Whence is it that this singular and unnatural change is taking place? Because that on women are imposed the duty and burden of supporting their husbands and family, a perversion as it were of nature, which has the inevitable effect of introducing into families disorder, insubordination and conflict....
>
> No, Sir, these sources of mischief must be dried up; every public consideration demands such an issue; the health of the females; the care of their families; their conjugal and parental duties; the comfort of their homes; the decency of their lives; the rights of their husbands; the peace of society; and the laws of God.[28]

The thoroughly interwoven mix of all the themes deemed necessary to the established social and moral order makes more understandable the fear and trepidation provoked by even the possibility that one of those constituent parts could be undermined and the whole edifice crumble. The issue of infanticide, however, did not provoke such fears.

Infanticide

The visible Victorian child was vulnerable and weak – the more dependent and innocent the more influential the image – but that factor alone cannot explain 'the discovery' of infanticide and the successful passage of the Infant Life Protection Act 1872 with its apparent focus on children when they are most dependent on parents. What the campaigners saw as seriously wrong were the births and deaths of infants which took place in very particular circumstances where regulation posed no serious challenge to the autonomy of the 'normal' family. According to the supporters of the legislation, babies needed protection against the immoral behaviour of those women – often single and unmarried – who left their (illegitimate) babies with 'baby farmers',[29] and also against the commercial nurses themselves. Those who opposed the original Bill that was placed before Parliament did so because it would also have caught in its net nurses in manufacturing districts who took children for the day, in other words, childminders who took in children of parents living in the type of unit defined as 'a family'. This would, as the National Society for Women's Suffrage expressed it, 'interfere in a most mischievous and oppressive way with domestic arrangements' (Pinchbeck and Hewitt, 1973, p. 617).[30] Therefore, pressure from women to preserve their traditional authority over 'mothering' gained strength from, and further buttressed, notions of family autonomy:

> The responsibility for the child in infancy as in later life, lies with [parents], and we emphatically deny that the State has any right to dictate to them the way it shall be fulfilled...the State should forbear to limit their perfect freedom in this, as in all matters connected with the rearing and maintaining of families.
> (The Committee for Amending the Law in Points where it is Injurious to Women, quoted in Pinchbeck and Hewitt, 1973, p. 618)

As a result, the Bill was limited in its scope to those children under one year old who were 'boarded out' for more than twenty-four hours.[31] In this campaign the construction of the enemy of children had been successfully confined to those who did not live in normal families. The prevalent morality still did not allow of it being defined as seriously wrong for 'normal' parents to use childminders whose standards of care might be seriously deficient.

Moral abuse: the delinquent child

The focus on the factory child and the minded/fostered baby had generally not required prosecutions against parents. Parents continued to be seen as the protectors, not the enemies, of children. Constructing the child as a victim of a known evil such as parental cruelty was insufficient if intervention threatened the dominant moral system. Something more was required: a threat to the moral system itself – an evil within the system emanating from the family unit that was greater than the threat posed by intervening in that family. This indeed occurred when parents were constructed as 'wicked' *specifically* because they were making their children wicked.[32] In other words, the image of the child was of one who was the victim of the parent, not because of physical and emotional harm done to him, but because of the moral evil inflicted on the child. In this sense constructing the child as evil does not, of itself, bar that child from victim status, because that evil is not the child's fault: innocence is imputed to him because his depravity is a result of his deprivation of proper paternal moral authority and control, and because that depravity is no longer seen as unchangeable.[33] The harm that the child is being protected from is the possibility that the child will be made permanently evil. As a result it became morally acceptable that the father who is not exerting proper moral control over his children should forfeit his paternal rights to control those children.

This shift in thinking about morality occurred over a number of years: major philanthropic societies with programmes to respond to juvenile criminality (or the risk of it) had been formed in 1788 and 1815 but parliamentary Bills based on their programmes failed in the 1820s (see Dingwall *et al.*, 1984, p. 214ff.). The social anxiety which acted to quicken the pace of the moral shift was the fact that the 1840s was a period of political instability. As the historian Kitson-Clarke states, '[Industrialization] had brought insecurity to all: by 1840 the bounding prosperity which the new industry had conferred had largely disappeared' (Kitson-Clarke, 1962, p. 88). Recovery began in the 1850s but the events of the 1840s – Chartist agitation, revolutions in several European states in 1848, the repeal of the Corn Laws, the Irish famine and subsequent Irish immigration into England – had facilitated the idea that it was morally justifiable to intervene in the family to remove children deemed at risk of (re-)offending, and to send such children to industrial schools for training. Similarly, convicted young offenders were seen to need reformatories – to compensate for the lack of moral training by their parents – rather than penal establishments. The shift was also justified in relation to the moral health of the abuser: 'The evil was as much the spiritual harm which befell the abusers as the physical or moral damage sustained by their victims' (Dingwall *et al.*, 1984, p. 218).

What this shift led to was a series of Industrial School Acts, 1857–1880,[34] to save children from being taught to be immoral in their families or on the streets, and to impose substitute parental discipline. Such schools could be eligible for grants from public funds. Similarly the Youthful Offenders Act 1854[35] made reformatory schools an alternative to adult prisons and houses of correction for juvenile offenders, and gave the voluntary societies who established and managed reformatories powers of compulsion over such children. This moral shift by the 1850s did not, however, justify the removal of children who had been physically abused by their parents: the fear of causing moral harm to the family by intervention weighed more heavily in the balance than the evil of parental cruelty.

What moral agenda explains the success of the cruelty campaigns in the 1880s?

> There is some dispute about the background to the anti-cruelty movement...
>
> (Dingwall *et al.*, 1984, p. 218)

The moral system of the 1850s to 1870s allowed no moral justification for intervention in the family against physical cruelty. When Dingwall *et al.* refer to the 'neglected continuities' between the campaign for factory laws and the campaign against family cruelty (Dingwall *et al.*, 1984, p. 218) they give a misleading impression. Certainly there were continuities of personnel in campaigns to prevent animal and child cruelty[36] but attention to these 'slack resources' (of 'spare' campaigners) sheds light only on how, technically, reform could be accomplished, not on how, morally, it became a social and political possibility. Morally, thinking in regard to the balancing of evils could be transformed in two ways: by a reduction in the moral authority of the traditional Victorian family; and by an increase in the 'volume' of evil which child abuse signified. The latter possibility has been refuted in so far as it relies on a false assumption that domestic violence was not seen as 'wrong' until the 1880s. However, the physical condition of children had become more visible (to the state's teachers and inspectors) since the 1870 Education Act, which led to the setting up of 'Board' (i.e. state) elementary schools.[37] 'Unsocialized' children were also more visible to other parents: 'The rakings of the human cesspool are brought into the school room and mixed up with your children....Childish innocence is very beautiful; but the bloom is soon destroyed.'[38]

As regards the former possibility, Behlmer's thesis is that respect for family integrity and paternal authority was still widespread and strong in the 1880s, and so the reason for the growth in the acceptability of intervention against parental cruelty has to be found elsewhere (Behlmer, 1982, ch. 3).[39] He provides evidence that belief in the 'sanctity of the home' was not weakening, citing literature on moral improvement in the later Victorian period which places the home at the centre of social and religious life. In 1849 John Ruskin had written, 'Our God is a household God as well as a heavenly one. He has an altar in every man's dwelling.'[40] In 1883 similar sentiments were still being published:

> Estimate the healing, comforting, purifying, elevating influence which is ever flowing from the fountain, and you will understand the sacred ministry of the home to the higher culture of mankind. It is a mighty restraint of the selfish passions. It is the centrifugal force which continually widens the orbit of life, and bears us into the light of distant suns.[41]

Indeed, the furore over the Education (Provision of Meals) Act 1906, twenty-three years after the above was written, testifies to the continuing strength of the belief in the moral importance of family autonomy. The Charity Organisation Society, for example, denounced the proposal in its report, 'The Better Way of Assisting School Children'.[42]

> It is better, in the interests of the community, to allow...the sins of the parents to be visited on the children, than to impair the principle of the solidarity of the family and run the risk of permanently demoralising large numbers of the population by the offer of free meals to their children.[43]

Instead, an understanding of how changes in perceptions of the moral framework became possible in the 1880s must focus on the social anxiety and the national moral crisis. First, from 1875 onwards, as in the decade before the passing of the first Industrial Schools Act, an economic recession led to perceptions of social and political instability. These social anxieties should not be underestimated. Historically, recessions had been accompanied by riots (e.g. in the 1810s and 1840s) and the 1880s themselves saw popular disturbances.

This social anxiety was also again linked to specific fears about urbanization. As Hendrick points out,[44] 'There was the "condition of England" question, first raised in the 1830s and 1840s, and rediscovered in the 1880s' (Hendrick, 1994, p. 50). The worst excesses of early urbanization had been ameliorated by legislation about housing, sanitation and public health but the increased geographical segregation of the rich and the poor which had occurred by the 1880s meant that the poorest lived in slums far removed from the dwellings of the rich: the 'distant' urban masses were more frightening than known neighbours. A later development (by the end of the century) feeding into this preexistent fear was eugenics (see Behlmer, 1982, p. 204). The result was that the urban poor perceived as a threat became labelled as 'a race apart', as 'the submerged tenth', and the areas of the United Kingdom in which they lived were referred to as 'Darkest England'.[45]

Anxiety was also engendered because of a relatively sudden loss of faith in 'progress'. Environmental measures had been passed in the belief that such legislation, given time, would 'solve' the social problems. It appeared that they would not. As a result, 'The environmentalism which had such an influence over social reform in mid-century began to give way again to a revived evangelicalism which emphasised depravity rather than deprivation' (Cox, 1996, p. 149). There was a sense that change must occur: 'We have made for ourselves strange gods, and we live in a state of transition to a yet unknown order', wrote Escott in 1881 in his introduction to *England: Its People, Polity and Pursuits*.[46]

These various social and political anxieties prompted the construction of intervention in the family as a lesser evil than undermining the entire moral framework of society which is what might happen unless selected families were regulated. The moral role of the family – feeding as it did into religion, social order, the health of a democracy and, therefore, the economic and political well-being of the country – became too important to leave to the family. A gradual reconstruction of the particular moral order to which the Victorians had been committed had occurred sufficiently by the end of the 1880s for the 'undisciplined' family (in which child abuse could happen and criminality could be encouraged) to be perceived as one which produced a moral imperative to intervene in that family.[47] Where life in particular families was not in practice sacred and moral, whether its immorality was evidenced by moral or physical abuse of children, it was no longer deemed to carry moral authority:

> The cruelties he warned against were unseen,...and public feeling resented any invasion of what was considered the sanctity of the home. To change this feeling it was necessary to show how little of the sacredness of family life existed among the more depraved, and the manner in which a man exercised his right to do what he would with his own.
>
> (Said of Benjamin Waugh, the congregational minister who became honorary secretary of the London Society for the Prevention of Cruelty to Children in Tuckwell, 1894)[48]

This process of focusing on how moral authority was exercised was one which absorbed, and was accelerated by, a redefining of Christian duty in relation to children. The 1886 NSPCC tract, *The Child of the English Savage*, added a particular gloss on the innocence of childhood: 'of all [God's] creatures [the child] is the most like Himself in its early purity, beauty, brightness and innocence' and so, by harming a child the Christian failed in his religious duty (Behlmer 1982, p. 87).

The general anxiety that moral structures were failing and that drastic action was necessary for the greater good allowed for a rebalancing of evils. The outcome of this rebalancing was never a foregone conclusion: the draft anti-cruelty Bill produced by the London SPCC in 1886 did not receive Home Office sponsorship; the first Bill presented to parliament in August 1888 met extensive opposition and was withdrawn despite the fact that the NSPCC did not support it because it was too weak a measure; the eventually successful Bill was sponsored by Mundella in February 1889 but, when passed, incorporated amendments.[49] Nevertheless, agitation did culminate in the Act for the Prevention of Cruelty to and Better Protection of Children in 1889. The NSPCC, in its report for 1895–6, looking back to the passage of that Act, said that 'it was nothing less than a national education which was undertaken...it was a crusade primarily to the intellect of the nation, preaching the existence and magnitude of the work to be done for needlessly suffering children'. When the Act was strengthened in further legislation in 1894, Lord Herschell, speaking in the House of Lords on the Bill, said 'there was not a few who at that time entertained some apprehensions with regard to entrusting powers so large – fears were expressed lest it might involve so much interference with parental control as to lead to dangerous results'.[50]

Later legislation in relation to child welfare and protection depended for its success on the same moral balancing exercise, though, as mentioned above, the social and political anxiety was heightened by a belief that 'The problem of the child is the problem of the race';[51] that

> Children thus hungered, thus housed, and thus left to grow up as best they can without being fathered or mothered, are not, educate them as you will, exactly the most promising material for the making of the future citizens and rulers of the Empire.
>
> (Booth, 1890, pp.65–6)

Lord Rosebery's call for a party of 'National Efficiency' was based on this belief that 'in the rookeries and slums which still survive, an imperial race cannot be reared'.[52] This fear increased at the time of the Boer War in England. To quote Spargo:

> In England the high infantile mortality has occasioned much alarm and caused forth much agitation. There is a world of pathos and rebuke in the grim truth that the knowledge that it is becoming increasingly difficult to get suitable recruits for the army and navy has stirred the nation in a way that the fate of the children themselves and their inability to become good and useful citizens could not do....No figures can adequately represent the meaning of this phase of the problem which has been so picturesquely named 'race suicide'. Only by gathering them all into one vast throng would it be possible to conceive vividly the immensity of this annual slaughter of the babies in a Christian land.
>
> (Spargo, [1906] 1969, pp. 9 and 10)

The concerns of the Edwardians, therefore, moved on from parental cruelty to issues of child poverty, education, hygiene and diet, but these new moral agendas for the early twentieth century cannot be pursued within the confines of this chapter.

Conclusion

Victorians campaigning for the welfare of children were driven by two sets of moral needs: needs stemming from their own personal and political anxieties, and also the perceived needs of selected children. For much of the century their motivation to improve the morality and personal responsibility of the poor and their children was religious. As late as 1890, William Booth, for example, in a chapter entitled 'On the verge of the abyss', asserted, 'at the risk of being misunderstood', that 'it is primarily and mainly for the sake of saving the soul that I seek the salvation of the body'. By the end of the century religious duty was joined by social guilt as a motivation for action. Simey, in her analysis of philanthropy in nineteenth-century Liverpool, has referred to the period 1875 to 1890 as one of 'Personal Service', when '[t]his sense of guilt was a new element in the relationship between rich and poor' (Simey, 1951).[53]

With these moral imperatives to act the campaigners designated particular harms to children – cruelty by the owners of factories, mines and baby nurseries, by single mothers and by fathers of delinquent children – as wrongs which required state-backed action at least partly because the morals of the children were also at risk. Intervention to prevent and punish physical cruelty required, therefore, a very radical shift in thinking. Parents themselves had to be seen as the enemies of children and the state, and voluntary organizations seen as their saviours. Such a shift in thinking has had far-reaching consequences for twentieth-century family policy. Once it had become possible to label particular parents as the source of the harm suffered by their child, then the way was open for other harms to justify not only intervention in the family but also the rescue of children from other sources of harm. Despite the refocusing on parental responsibility in the last quarter of the twentieth century, there is no longer social and governmental reticence in blaming parents for harms inflicted on, and by, their children.

Notes

1 The context for this quotation is an introductory chapter on 'The Child in History' and, in particular, a discussion of historical perceptions of children, rather than the experiences of children in different historical periods.

2 For further discussion, see Tosh (1995), p. 114.

3 So, for example, Carson (1974) analysed the genesis of the nineteenth-century Factory Acts through a study of the employer interest in productivity and healthier employees. Feminist historians looked at the role of male trade unions in seeking reform of working conditions for women and children, which would, as a side-product, increase the male wage and improve the terms of employment for men.

4 For further discussion, see Tosh (1995), pp. 178–9.

5   At its simplest, a discourse is a social process in which, through
        language (used in its broadest sense to include all semiotic systems)
        we make sense of the world around us, but also the process by which
        the world makes sense to us.

                     (Cox, 1996, p. 6, referring to O'Sullivan *et al.*, 1994)

6 Becker's research looked at responses to marijuana users, dealing specifically with moral crusaders/entrepreneurs in ch. 8; Gusfield researched the
   Prohibition movement in the USA, discussing 'status politics' in ch. 7,
   where he focuses on the meaning inherent in political action and
   discourse.
7 For example, Eekelaar *et al.* (1982); Dingwall *et al.* (1984, 1995).
8 The first wave of evangelical reformers – from the end of the eighteenth
   century – were, as Hendrick points out, 'the foremost in an appreciation
   of the importance of childhood'. In particular, he quotes Hannah More, a
   founder of the Sunday School movement: 'Where are the half-naked, poor,
   forlorn, wretched, ignorant creatures we used to find lying about on
   Sunday...?' (Hendrick, 1994, p. 8).
9 Referred to by Behlmer (1982), p. 3 and Cunningham (1995), p. 143.
   The latter text excerpts a verse of that poem, the last two lines of which
   are: 'They are weeping in the playtime of the others, / In the Country of
   the free'.
10 Originally published in the USA and reprinted in 1969.
11 This elision of victim and voiceless statuses is not simply a product of
   Victorian sentimentality: those pressing for 'rights' for victims of crime in
   the 1980s and 1990s have also constructed the lack of voice as a key
   element of victim status. See, for example, Sarat (1997).
12 *Memoirs of the Life and Writings of Michael Thomas Sadler, M.P.; F.R.S.; &c.*,
   337/379 1842, excerpted on p. 102 of Ward (1970).
13 The phrase used by Douglas Jerrold, one of the founders of *Punch*, in 1840
   to describe factory children. Quoted by Cunningham (1995), p. 144.
14 This is not an entirely accurate statement in that the 'sending away' of
   children, of all classes, to work in the households of relatives or strangers
   was a common occurrence in earlier centuries, notably the sixteenth and
   seventeenth. (E.g. see Pinchbeck and Hewitt 1969 pp. 25–30 regarding
   upper-class girls and pp. 223–59 regarding the Poor Law apprenticeship
   system.) The novelty is in the extent and nature of this out-of-family
   working.
15 In fact, the numbers of people living in the countryside may have
   increased rather than declined in the early nineteenth century and the
   numbers of people living in towns were still lower than those in rural
   areas by the 1851 census (Kitson-Clarke, 1961, pp. 117–18). The 'fact'
   underlying the sense of unease was that the numbers in towns had
   increased comparatively quickly. For example, the population of
   Manchester and Salford rose from 95,000 in 1801 to 238,000 in 1831
   (Pinchbeck and Hewitt, 1973, p. 389).
16 See, for example, Cohen (1972).
17 It should not be forgotten, however, that there was considerable cruelty to
   children in the 'old' workplace, that is in agriculture, especially with the

development of the gang labour system in the second quarter of the nineteenth century (see Pinchbeck and Hewitt, 1973, pp. 391–5).

18 See Cunningham (1995), pp. 138–45.

19 Jane Addams, an American philanthropist born in 1859, wrote: 'let us know the modern city in its weakness and wickedness, and then seek to rectify and purify it' (quoted in Platt, 1969, p. 96).

20 See the article by Bar-On (1997) analysing research done in Ghana, Namibia and Zambia.

21 Referred to by Dingwall *et al.* (1984), p. 219.

22 Quoted on p. 622 of Pinchbeck and Hewitt (1973).

23 Both quoted in C.L. Mowat (1961), pp. 21 and 71 respectively.

24 An impression given by Pinchbeck and Hewitt (1969), pp. 302–6.

25 I am grateful to Stephen Cretney for suggesting this perspective: *CFLQ* Seminar, All Souls Oxford, 1 July 1997.

26 Pinchbeck and Hewitt do however refer to a 'radical group' who campaigned from the 1860s for state action to break the link between the employment of mothers and the early death of their children (1973, pp. 358–9).

27 On 15 March in the debate in committee on the Factories Bill dealing with hours of labour in factories.

28 Quoted on pp. 68–9 of Cairns (1965).

29 See Behlmer (1982), ch. 2 for a very good account of the context of this Act.

30 Their argument was that, whilst they approved of licensing, they did not feel it right to compel parents to employ only licensed minders.

31 This age limit was not raised to five years until 1897 and to seven years until 1908.

32 When discussing the Maloney Report of 1927 Dingwall *et al.* note the same concern: 'The neglect that is being talked about, however, is not a want of physical care but an attention to the control and moral education of children' (1984, p. 216).

33 To quote Cunningham again, 'Children were thought to be unformed enough to be saveable' (1995, p. 135).

34 Industrial schools had been set up since the eighteenth century both under the Poor Law and by charitable bodies, though compulsion to attend could generally be only on the children of families claiming poor relief or on orphans. For a fuller discussion, see Pinchbeck and Hewitt (1973), pp. 530–2.

35 See Pinchbeck and Hewitt (1973), ch. 16 for a full discussion, including details of the 1854 Act at pp. 476–7. By 1859 fifty reformatory schools had been established.

36 See Behlmer (1982), p. 67ff.

37 See Hendrick (1994), pp. 29–33 and, p. 50. An example of how the state acquired information about its children can be found in the Final Report of the Royal Commission on the Elementary Education Acts (1888, c. 5495) which noted in Part IV under the heading 'Physical Training': 'care however must always be taken in applying such training to delicate and underfed children'.

38 W. Booth (1890), ch. VIII: 'The children of the lost', pp. 63–4.

39 Though not directly relevant to this analysis, it is worth noting that Behlmer also argues that there was no economic explanation in that children were of diminishing economic importance in that period: in 1851 they constituted 6.9 per cent of the workforce whereas in 1881 only 4.5 per cent (1982, p. 46).

40 J. Ruskin, *The Seven Lamps of Architecture*, first edition, p. 184, 1849, quoted in Himmelfarb (1995), p. 56.

41 J.B. Brown, *The Home: In its Relation to Man and Society*, p. 47, 1883, quoted in Behlmer (1982), p. 46.

42 See Mowat (1961), pp. 74–5 and pp. 154–5.

43 Quoted by Pinchbeck and Hewitt (1973), p. 358.

44 In the context of arguing for the 'condition of England' as the most influential factor influencing the construction of child abuse as 'a major social disease' in the 1880s.

45 General William Booth of the Salvation Army produced a book of evidence about the poor entitled *In Darkest England and the Way Out* and referred to the population under scrutiny as 'the submerged tenth'.

46 An entry in Beatrice Webb's Diary for November 1886 reveals the same questioning of long-held beliefs: 'There are times when one loses all faith in laisser-faire and would suppress the poison at all regards for it eats the life of the nation.' Webb was referring to her East End of London research and, in particular, to the 'poison' of 'drink' (quoted in ch. 6 of Webb *My Apprenticeship* 1926).

47 As Cox notes, 'the bourgeoisie as a class was one that always sensed a threat from within, in terms of a failure of its own cultural reproduction, and from without, through the external threat of mass society' (Cox, 1996, p. 200).

48 Gertrude Tuckwell, *The State and its Children*, p. 127, 1894, quoted in Pinchbeck and Hewitt (1973), pp. 622–3.

49 See Behlmer (1982), ch. 4 for details. The amendments which were accepted to promote the passage of the Act were that the age limit for jurisdiction under the Act was lowered from sixteen to fourteen for boys and that less tight restrictions were imposed on street trading by children.

50 Hansard, 1894, xxiv, col. 1609, quoted in Pinchbeck and Hewitt (1973), p. 629.

51 H.D. Chapin in *The Theory and Practice of Infant Feeding*, quoted in Spargo. Spargo enlarges on this statement 'the physician traces the weakness and disease of the adults to defective nutrition in early childhood; the penologist traces moral perversion to the same cause; the pedagogue finds the same explanation for his failures' (Spargo, [1906] 1969, pp. 2–3).

52 Taken from a speech by Rosebery in 1901 and quoted in Semmel (1960), p. 62.

53 The resolution produced in November 1883 to announce the intention of setting up a Fabian Society said that its ultimate aim would be 'the reconstruction of society in accordance with the highest moral possibilities'. Quoted in M. Cole, *The Story of Fabian Socialism*, London: Heinemann, 1961.

4 Liberalism or distributional justice?

The morality of child welfare laws

Terry Carney[1]

Introduction

Child welfare is a subset of national welfare policies. As with the welfare state, it has taken many turnings as social, economic and political values and priorities have altered. Childhood is a social construct, a product of the culture of the time (James and Jenks, 1996, pp. 317–18). Not only has it changed over time, but various groups of professionals may interpret (or 'read') childhood and children's needs differently at given times (King, 1981), or according to different cultural values and national perspectives (comparative international examples of laws and systems of administration may differ radically from British experience, for example). This chapter is unashamedly eclectic and ambitious in its sweep of comparative material. It locates itself more in political theory than may be comfortable for some historians, philosophers, or lawyers. It is anchored differently from other contributions in this collection, and it offers a more open-textured narrative. In this it too reflects the cultural forces which, it is argued, have shaped thinking about our subject matter of children, law, morality and distributional justice. Each of which terms is notoriously slippery. All are 'fat' words: they conceal many (sometimes even incompatible) shades of meaning.[2]

Until the mid-nineteenth century the very idea of discussing the intersection of the terms 'childhood' and 'welfare' would have met with puzzlement. Little distinction was made between adolescent children and adults because of their importance in pre-industrial agrarian family production.[3] 'Innocence' was rather the badge of young children (see Piper, Chapter 3, pp. 35–6). Welfare too was a very different category to the contemporary understanding of the term, in several ways. Welfare was a private or philanthropic responsibility rather than a state function (Finlayson, 1994). Moreover, poverty, child neglect and juvenile crime (and even health), were all closely intertwined in the public mind (including public debate and policy-making); and each was infused by a robust and unforgiving form of religious moralism. Social problems were attributed to such things as a person's lack of moral fibre, alcoholism, thriftlessness or criminal propensity. Evil was fashionable and it came in several shapes and sizes.

Changing contours of childhood and child welfare

Changing moral pictures of childhood

Widespread concern emerged, and strong public campaigns were waged against the exploitation of child labour during the early part of the industrial revolution. A combination of factors such as moral outrage and a rising demand for a better trained workforce in the latter half of the nineteenth century led to enactment of compulsory education and child labour laws,[4] though pattern and complexity varied from place to place.[5] Currency was given to Rousseau's ideas about the malleability, innocence and fragility of childhood.[6] Around the turn of the century, social movements sought to save children from the inhumanity (and contamination) of the adult system.[7] Mary Carpenter won support for her industrial and reform schools as an alternative to adult correction.[8] In Australia, where child protection services became a state (not local authority) responsibility early on, this was followed by widespread resort to placement of neglected children (called statutory state wards) into foster care and apprenticeships, once residential institutions lost their gloss.[9] Childhood innocence was now to be immunized against the external threat posed by forces of social corruption (cf. Rousseau). A moral floor was constructed in the hope of keeping children on a plane higher than the depths of depravity or degradation to which adult mortals might fall. The space occupied by childhood had become 'innocence enshrined' (James and Jenks, 1996, p. 315).

Hard on the heels of this (in the late nineteenth century) came the moves to consolidate these conceptual gains through establishment of separate 'children's courts' – first in America, closely followed by Australia and Canada. Britain was something of an exception, both in its tardy response and its disinclination to break with a mainly 'criminal justice' paradigm; and, as King (1981) observes, not only was child neglect left mainly in the hands of local government, but the rise of 'welfare' approaches may overstate and oversimplify debates.[10] The assumption underpinning the new children's courts was of a 'defective socialisation of children and that in order to rehabilitate them they [required to be] treated and cared for in a personal manner' (Murray, 1985, p. 75; also Dingwall *et al.*, 1984, p. 207). It was the image of the child as being vulnerable and in need which was the basis for state action; the cause of that need, and even the form in which it manifested itself, was irrelevant. Hence the blurring of distinctions between child neglect and child delinquency; the civil orientation of the court; the interdisciplinary focus on the therapeutic potential of the helping professions; and the appropriation into the children's courts of the sentiments underlying the paternal jurisdiction of English courts of Chancery in their 'ward of court' role.[11] This more optimistic (indeed idealistic) vision of the early twentieth century originated in ideas of the moral and social *perfectibility* of the young.

This had its counterpart in responding to delinquency too. The young were to receive different treatment from adults *irrespective* of whether their degree of moral culpability was the same (as would be the case with say a premeditated major crime by an older adolescent). Generally, that culpability was diminished, either by lessened capacity to form a moral judgement (the basis of the *doli incapax* rule for children under fourteen, which precludes conviction unless the prosecution proves moral understanding), or by virtue of immaturity and a presumed greater responsiveness to measures of moral rehabilitation. The point is that the essence of the argument shifted. Instead of responding to the moral (and social or other) content of the criminal *deed* which brought a person before the court (the logic of the 'tariff' basis for sentencing adults), the focus was instead on the psychological or other *needs* of the delinquent. The language of therapy became dominant at the expense of the language of moral accountability (O'Connor, 1997).[12]

The idea that some children do not commit violent crime, and at times horrible acts, was always a myth of course (Richards, 1997, p. 64). However, until recently, rare events such as murder by a child, escaped the 'high frenzy' of close public scrutiny (Metcalf, 1994). This is not to say that public imaginations were not titillated, but such events did not attract a tabloid 'feeding frenzy'. It is argued here that this was because the dominant legal (and media) narratives were those of innocence and human perfectibility. It would be naïve to think that because Britain did not budge far from a classical criminal model public opinion mimicked that stance; or that Scotland, in its warm embrace of 'needs' philosophy through its Children's Hearing approach introduced in 1969, was somehow a 'land apart' compared to public opinion in England and Wales.

Whatever the reading of the public mood may be (and the 'philosophy' which it encapsulates), it cannot be disputed that in times of social tension youth commonly becomes one of the community's scapegoats. This was true during the dislocation associated with the gold rushes in Australia; just as it was in the US and Canada.[13] It remains no less true today, whether we turn to Australia (White *et al.*, 1991), Canada (Baron and Hartnagel, 1996), or Britain (Morrison, 1994, p. 56). The patina on the more morally uplifting visions of childhood has been rubbed back. They have been eroded by rising levels of general community anxiety about static living standards, lessening of the certitudes of life, growing disparities of wealth, and rising unemployment. The baser social instincts are again revealed, as they were during Poor Law times, including a revival of interest in Puritan notions of intrinsic badness (or sin), and greater stress on personal accountability.

This introduces a sharp and troubling dissonance of conflicting narratives, a break from the dominant influence of many of the assumptions of the child saving philosophy which shaped both policy and social attitudes over much of the twentieth century. Prominent media coverage of events such as the murder in Britain of two-year-old James Bulger by two ten-year-olds counterpoises two 'iconocologically irreconcilable' images (James and Jenks, 1996, p. 320). As Diduck argues in Chapter 8, such events represent the disjunction between socially connective (mothering) notions of 'care and welfare' for children, and the new settings of children's lives (in which they are, for example, consumers, occupiers of public space and rights bearers). One possibility is that the connective 'moral and ethical relations' carry the day against weak 'justice' protections: children may be demonized and thereby excluded from enjoyment of social, civil or political society. Another possibility, also illustrated by the Bulger case, is that children may be reconceptualized as adults, without making any concessions (Diduck, Chapter 8, pp. 129–32).

The Bulger case similarly became a symbolic point of 'connotative resonance' for several wider discourses, each with its origins in rising social insecurity (Hay, 1995, p. 217). Such moral panics gain their momentum from their symbolic representation of a link between such things as the 'the threats posed by the dynamism and flux of modernity' and 'nostalgia for an idealised past' (where maternal responsibility, moral sanctity and stability of the family unit, and clear male authority existed: *ibid.*, p. 199). In such cases it serves to unify twin themes of the 'threat posed by juvenile criminality', with subversion of 'otherwise "innocent" youth through the breakdown of the "traditional" moral family unit' (*ibid.*, p. 217). A new 'narrative' (or story) has come to replace the old. It is a moral narrative of personal or family responsibility, rather than a social narrative which looks for explanations in the quality and scale of public sector provision such as child care services, schools, or family and social services. Diduck in this book recognizes the gravity of the challenge posed, arguing that it calls for a radical redrawing of boundaries of childhood and justice, in order to recontextualize children within a 'more nuanced' conception of justice.

This contested policy narrative of childhood and justice is matched by similar changes in the philosophies underpinning different legislative models of child welfare.

The rise and partial decline of child saving policies

The late 1890s witnessed the emergence in America, Canada and Australia of what is termed the 'child saving' movement,[14] modified and muted in Britain by the strength of religious endorsement of the 'family' and by the fillip given to reform by insecurities generated by economic recession. This movement had several features. It drew a clear line between adulthood and childhood; it marked acceptance of childhood as a more extended and distinctive stage of social and individual *development*; and it gave prominence to the social ceremonies which mark that transition to adulthood. One of its by-products was that child welfare was recognized as a distinctive field of policy, with its own rationale. That rationale was strongly infused with principles of state paternalism, whereas liberalism and personal accountability were the watchwords emblematic of the adult system. The associated invention of a separate structure of courts and departments of state charged with protection of children, simply provided the channel for expression of that rationale.

Over the course of the twentieth century, state child welfare policy has oscillated markedly.[15] At first it was influenced most by ideas of classical nineteenth-century utilitarian liberalism: intervention into the zone of choice and autonomy of action of the family unit was based on a clear showing of damage to the public (an offence) or harm to the child (child neglect). Britain apart (where the trend was muted), this was then replaced by a greater emphasis on ideas of state paternalism. This latter was expressed in the guiding philosophy of children's courts established in America, where the movement reached its zenith, as illustrated by its use of the metaphor of a children's court as equivalent to a 'father' dealing with a child in 'his' study. This same approach, but in lesser measure was also applied in the children's courts of Canada and Australia. Children were portrayed as innocents to be protected against the corrupting influences of weak families, moral danger, criminal influences and poverty. Here crime and neglect were seen more as products of the context in which a child was raised than results of the individual moral fault of either the child or their family. Intervention was grounded in establishing a child's *need* or likely *future* needs, rather than clear *proof* of *present harm*.

Certainly, North America embraced paternalism more warmly than did say Australia and Scotland (and more so than in England and Wales). Even so, the zenith of state paternalism has long since passed. Paternalism does still remain as a significant influence over contemporary child welfare policies, but its excesses have been checked by a re-emphasis on the need for proof, proportionality and realism of therapeutic ambitions in the fields of child protection and delinquency. It has also been reined in by international recognition of children's rights, culminating in the 1989 United Nations Convention on the Rights of the Child.[16]

During the 1970s and 1980s most common law jurisdictions witnessed an ebbing away of policies of child protection based on judgements made about children's alleged 'needs', whether social or moral. Those policies were replaced by interventions grounded in the notion of tangible risk of significant 'harms' to the child or young person. As regards morality, the statute books were cleansed of the capacity to find that a child was 'exposed to moral danger' or 'likely to lapse into a career of vice and crime'; both of which were legacies of the Poor Law of England and, as such, had attracted criticism both for their open-ended character and their liability to reflect narrow readings of accepted cultural values (O'Connor, 1997). Outside the moral sphere, this change to a 'current harms' policy was made because, as the Australian Law Reform Commission documented (Australian Law Reform Commission (ALRC), 1981), needs proved elusive, cold empirical evaluations of state intervention found that it often compounded rather than alleviated needs, and interventions were often disproportionate in both their scale and their duration. Levels of state resourcing tended to ebb on the same tide, however, leaving many children and families with less support than they may have needed.

Moreover, the previous sense of threat and evil experienced by previous generations did not die away entirely. In newly settled countries in particular, young people, as we have seen, have been one of the first groups to be demonized when the pace of social change and economic dislocation posed too great a threat to the social dominance, economic interests and social values of prior waves of settlement.[17] Back in fashion at such times is the grammar of individual account- ability by children for their actions, of family 'fault' rather than social responsibility, and of the 'moral maturity' of young people in place of diminished capacity. The present is such a time.

Changes in the character of the state have also been evident. These are changes driven by the imperatives of economic rationalism, but infused with a new rationale – that of 'contractualism'. This is a ratio- nale very much at odds with the 'citizenship' explanation for conventional welfare state action.

Changing conceptions of the (welfare) state

Child welfare and 'citizenship' concepts

Citizenship concepts theorized by political scientists and social policy analysts (among many others) have provided a powerful tool not only for conceptualizing the welfare state, but also for drawing out distinc- tions both between 'active' and passive forms of state action, and between individual and collective expressions of welfare.[18] 'Social' citi- zenship, as portrayed by T.H. Marshall in a famous and much republished lecture first delivered in the late 1940s, was conceived as one of three interlocking sets of rights. The trilogy comprised both the previously recognized categories of 'civil' (legal process) and 'political process' rights (such as the franchise) which were successively consoli- dated during the eighteenth and nineteenth centuries in Britain. This was complemented by the set of 'social' rights emblematic of the twen- tieth-century welfare state.[19] Social citizenship, then, was the principal new 'good' conferred by the welfare state. This social right to full participation in society was elevated to equal importance with guaran- tees of political rights such as universal suffrage, or civil rights such as equality before the law.[20] If those rights are extended unconditionally, they constitute a 'status' or passive entitlement akin to the liberal institution of property (indeed, in North America, claims to welfare were conceptualized as 'new property' rights: Reich, 1964).[21] This analysis has been applied to child welfare too. Thus, even a rights sceptic such as O'Neill concedes the validity of *some* negative rights for children (1992, p. 32).[22]

However, social rights of citizenship can also be conceived as the ingredients necessary to found the 'activity' of social participation,[23] or in terms of what people *do* as distinct from what they *get* (Davidson, 1997). This overcomes the objection that when welfare is conceived of merely as a passive 'status' (see Moon, 1993), it fails to guarantee more than the basic necessities of life, leaving people at risk of social isolation in two ways: by ignoring their necessary social relationships, and by leaving them with a level of provision which fosters 'outsider' status. This critique, and the wider vision of active citizenship, may be applied to young people too.[24] This wider conception of social rights builds on two important elements of a traditional analysis of the welfare state – first, the recognition of the moral duty of the state to protect vulnerable people irrespective of fault; and second, compliance with the principle of the rule of law (that entitlements should not be at the whim of the state or be subject to arbitrary change). However the active version of citizenship is not unproblematic, and may be too vague and woolly an idea to take us very far (Goodin and Le Grande, 1987, p. 12).

In the first place, it does not immunize against moral panic reactions. One of the most disturbing reactions to extreme and atypical situations such as the Bulger case, is that politicians may succumb to populist pressure to 'throw away the key', as the Home Secretary arguably did in this instance by fixing a fifteen-year non-release term.[25] Even in routine cases, ideas of active citizenship for the young must also be leavened by a realistic understanding of the challenges of the transition to adulthood, and of the role of culture and economic circumstances in defining its speed. Otherwise expectations of the young will be set at unrealistic levels.

Nor is this the only rub. Active citizenship may be code for opening the door to 'the visible hand of rulers who tell people what to do' (Dahrendorf, 1994, p. 13). It may go hand in hand with state withdrawal of responsibility for welfare provision, leaving vulnerable young people to the vagaries of the market, their 'family', and more personally accountable for their fate (Harris, 1993b, p. 206). This is particularly so under 'citizenship of contribution' formulations popularized by Conservative administrations in Britain.[26] Australian and American experience with 'work for the dole' initiatives is another indication of that trend. Australian government reforms removing unemployment benefits for young people (under twenty-one) not in full-time education or training, is yet another.

Active citizenship, then, is an imperfect benchmark. But it is notable for its endorsement of a state responsibility to foster the interests of (young) citizens in participating in the life of the community; a duty which *can* ground positive rights to such things as income support, housing, employment and training measures, but one which may not *necessarily* lead down a legal pathway which will guarantee such rights. Indeed, there is of course a respectable argument that law is entirely irrelevant, that it is a mistake to attempt to incorporate other dialogues into law, since law mangles and reconstitutes relationships in ways which alter original meanings.[27]

Short of this, there is a strong case for at least recognizing that, as contained in international instruments (such as the UN Convention) welfare 'rights' are expressed much more loosely, and are hedged with many more qualifiers, than are traditional civil rights (like freedom from torture). They serve more as rhetorical claims, sounding in the sphere of politics, than as rights statements awaiting easy conversion into legally secured entitlements.[28] As a consequence, traditional forms of 'prescriptive' legislation, and redress by way of judicial (or even administrative tribunal) adjudication may not be an ideal vehicle for their realization.

Yet it does not necessarily follow that law cannot express such entitlements in other, more 'relational' forms,[29] or that such entitlements cannot be adequately protected under more flexible, informal and mediated forms of review.[30] Tribunals (with lawyers in the minority) have been found to out-perform courts when dealing with substitute decision-making for instance (Carney and Tait, 1997). The positive entitlements envisioned by active citizenship participation need not remain mere weasel words whose realization lies outside the province of law. Rather it is the contraction of the state which may be the more significant inhibiting factor.

Child welfare in the 'contractualist' welfare state

Just as debate about social citizenship rights became a shorthand way of describing the rise of the postwar *bureaucratic* welfare state, so reflections on 'contractualism' may be seen as emblematic of its decline, and its transformation. Contractualism is a word which resonates with a return to individualism, both in greater reliance on individual provision than on state services or regulation, and in the return of contractual relations. This rise of 'contractualism', with its individualization of social relationships, is a feature of contemporary social policy.[31] Contractualism, as the term implies, injects ideas of private contract into the way the state relates to citizens (such as contracting out delivery of mental health or other services),[32] or as a precondition to gaining access to public benefits and services or to income security (which is also moving from 'status' to 'contract').[33]

It reflects a deliberate policy of withdrawing the state from its (Keynesian) regulatory oversight of such things as credit, trade and wage relations,[34] and is said to better accommodate new (so-called post-Fordist) forms of industrial production, the rise of globalization, and the more pluralist postmodern culture.[35] It permits the state to manifest itself in a greater variety of forms (it does not just make laws and deliver services) and in a greater variety of settings than it previously did (private entrepreneurs may take over state responsibilities for aged care, or the family may become an agent of state regulation). Commentators speak of this as the state becoming more 'differentiated'. In its contemporary form the state is now characterized by greater fragmentation, flexibility and sensitivity to markets.[36] The hallmarks of this situation include disaggregation, localization and variation in patterns of service provision.[37] Individual contractual agreements are becoming a prime way of achieving this within welfare. Privatization is also on the march in the related field of family law (Singer, 1992). This is a trend which has both negative and positive features.

On its more arid side is its association with a form of classical liberalism, where individual choice is a zone of 'negative' liberty from interference; moral responsibility is attributed to all actions; and state engineered distributional equality is not a valid goal. Contractualism necessarily dilutes the influence of rules or standards set by parliament, and expands the space for the exercise of either private discretion (as in much family law reform) or, in the case of welfare services, for the exercise of administrative discretion by public servants (or private contractors doing the bureaucrats' traditional work). This carries the potential of magnifying inequalities of power. Relationships are often expressed in loose, subjective language, and they are no longer transparent to public debate. Negotiation and compliance may be left to the parties, or private sector agencies (or to mediating agents). Any state oversight is unlikely to continue to follow Weberian ideas of objectivity, neutrality and arms-length administration. Private brokerage replaces governance by parliamentary rules and standards. Review by courts or tribunals may be withdrawn or rendered ineffective.[38]

In more positive vein, contractualism may bring benefits. In family law in recent times in Australia, Canada and America, state regulation (public ordering) has been open to the charge that its operation has often been sexist (implicitly stereotyping male and female roles), reinforcing of (male) hierarchy, and riven with dubious value assumptions such as female dependency (Singer, 1992, pp. 1532–3). Contractualism has also been advocated as a device to promote social participation by providing access to a wider range of social goods or entitlements (such as work: Pixley, 1993, pp. 11, 31); to replenish the mutuality of reciprocal relations between citizens and the state (Wilson, 1994, p. 53); and to inject greater flexibility and accountability (Nelken, 1987, pp. 209–12). One of these claimed benefits is the emphasis on tailoring the formation of 'self-regulated' social relationships (Yeatman, 1995, p. 132).

Contractualism, with its dismantling of public law in place of expansion in the spaces within which private ordering may take place, poses a particular difficulty for children, however. It is problematic enough for adults, but at least there is general acceptance of their capacity for autonomous action, and of the legal right to express that autonomy (unless contrary to the public interest or private welfare). As Yeatman observes, this leaves room to inject a feminist critique as a way of moderating the application of contractualism for adults. Adults can agree among themselves to adopt a 'combined ethic of care and empowerment' in place of contractualism's rampant individualism. This is a plausible gloss on contractualism as a policy for adults but it is not open as a way of moderating its application to children. This is because children's development of moral and decisional capacity is progressive (Morgan, 1986, pp. 181–95) and, traditionally, the law has been reluctant to attribute autonomy to the child (*ibid.*, pp. 163–74).

A solution for those unable to choose for themselves might be thought to lie in giving this mediating role to parents or other substitute decision-makers acting as 'trustees' of the interests of the child. Yeatman remains unconvinced by this. She argues that in practice the fidelity of the trust reposed in such parental or other 'carers' will be measured against sexist and individual-centred standards such as those of 'good' mothering (Yeatman, 1995, p. 135). Instead of injecting a counter-balancing ethic of care, grounded in a web of relationships negotiated between adult equals, contractualism as it applies to children will remain a private, individual space, one dominated by 'mothering' ideas which tend to reinforce the inferior status and power of women. In short, children and their (female) parental carers will continue to be disempowered by contractualism. While the traditional welfare role of public agencies of the state (e.g. child protection laws) is equally open to criticism that its vaunted 'best interests of the child' test is nothing more than an 'empty vessel' into which 'adult prejudices and perceptions' are poured (Rodham, 1973), at least this operates as a *public* space. Because it is a public space it has the attraction of being more contestable than is the privatized space implicit in contractualist policies for children.

The critical aspect of contractualism as it applies to children, then, is that there are damaging implications of the policy precisely because it *shifts* responsibilities from the public to the private (family) sectors without replicating the limited protections offered by public welfare, and without challenging the validity of that public/private divide (Woodhouse, 1993). In the case of adults, we have seen that it is conceivable that a more communal ethos can be agreed between individual citizens as a way of ameliorating contractualism without requiring its outright rejection. In the case of children, however, it is not possible to avoid the need to reconcile three sets of interests: those of the child, those of the family and those of the 'public'. Since children (and families) are not always self-sufficient, striking a balance between individualism and communitarianism necessarily raises questions about whether the answer is to be found by saying that support 'ought to come from family members, binding the individual', or whether it ought to come 'from the state, liberating the individual but binding the community' (Woodhouse, 1993, p. 512).[39] This is a tricky conundrum for contractualism. On the current evidence it is difficult to avoid the conclusion that more attention needs to be paid to finding ways of further *dissolving* the dichotomy between public and private spheres of action, such as by seeking creative ways of adapting the existing role and function of *public* agencies and services. This is the question to which we will now turn.

Postmodernism?

Various writers claim that contemporary social conditions call for more localized, open-textured, and 'responsive' settings for the application of policy. This is especially prominent in countries which have witnessed high levels of immigration, leading to much more heterogeneous (or 'multicultural') populations, with consequential changes to the public polity (Davidson, 1997). While mainly driven by other influences (globalization, technology, etc.) this has led countries such as America, Canada and Australia to give earlier attention to the implications of these global trends than may be the case in Britain or parts of Europe.

One possible response is to introduce a system giving much more scope for discretion (Simon, 1983). Under that scheme, social expectations (or 'values', p. 1224) would be very lightly sketched by the legislature as 'standards' (not rules) and their real content then supplied later by way of collegiate processes of professional officers and 'decentralised enforcement proceedings in which citizens participate' (Simon, 1983, p. 1242). Enforcing the adherence of administration to those expectations would rest with their ethical standards and professional culture.[40] This approach is less radical than it seems at first blush. The contraction of state child protection laws, from their wider 'preventive welfare' mandate to concentrate instead on tangible and immediate harms, certainly led to the vacation of ground previously occupied by public welfare agencies and services, leaving it free to be occupied in new ways – by the family; by voluntary self-help groups; or by professional social workers operating in the non-government sector. And it has been argued that England's experience with a wider 'welfare' role, such as through reliance on postnatal and health visitors, also depended on the forging of tacit understandings between the (professional and semi-professional) agents of the state and the families they worked with (Dingwall *et al.*, 1984). Given the shifts in juvenile justice policy, there have been significant changes in the proportionate reliance on family responsibility, philanthrophic and non-government services, professional discretion and state agency regulatory interventions (such as through the children's court).

The interest in placing much greater reliance on such new approaches than has been the case in the past stems from a couple of sources. First it recognizes that there may be some force in the iconoclasm characteristic of so-called 'postmodern' scholarship, a scholarship which questions the validity of traditional categories and boundaries.[41] Second, it re-engages philosophic (and socio-political) questions about liberty. It revisits what Erich Fromm, in his book *Fear of Freedom*, described as the distinction between freedom *from*, and freedom *to*; or as Berlin (1969) put it, the difference between negative and positive liberty (see Ferry, 1994, p. 294). As we have seen, positive liberty often rests in collective action that is expressed either by the state (in child protection or welfare services) or informally through 'community'. As the state has contracted (or been transformed), renewed interest has been generated in how positive liberty might be realized either outside the state (and law) or at least in its 'shadow'.[42]

One way in which this might be realized is by fostering what Handler (1988) calls a 'dialogic community'. This expression of interdependence may arise naturally outside the law (and traditional boundaries of the state), or it may arise in areas where discretions are provided: '[i]t asks: in these spaces, what are the conditions necessary for community?' (Handler, 1988, p. 1001). In either setting, it is plain that these conditions must include adequate guarantees against oppression from inequalities of power and subjection to hierarchy. Within child protection it must also deal with latent (or express) coercion, and the vulnerabilities which expose some children and some families to a need to engage with these services or agencies. As Foucault (1973) recognizes, these are the features which allow the state to extend its reach into apparently private spheres.

However, in situations of caring for the frail or vulnerable, the participatory 'dialogic community' only very rarely emerges, instead succumbing to forms of 'legal-bureaucratic' relationships. This may be attributed to over-dominance of the negative conceptions of rights enshrined by 'liberal legalism' (Handler, 1988, p. 1018). Additionally, the state may be overreaching itself or chasing the wrong (substantive) objectives when it would be better to focus on creating suitable processes (dialogic spaces),[43] or, as Teubner argues, on recognizing that the areas of interest may be self-governing and self-contained 'domains' with their own internal logic.[44]

These are important debates, but where do ethics and morality fit in? Populist stereotyping may inappropriately demonize children by stripping away the facade of 'innocence', or by seeking to correct their immorality.[45] Certainly it can be argued that it is right to resist repeating the errors of legislating such moral standards under the mounting pressure of public campaigns which have echoes of the 'moral crusades' of the late nineteenth century (see Piper, Chapter 3). We can sympathize too with Archard's plea to confine the definition of abuse justifying state intervention to serious breaches of 'core' values about which there is little disagreement, ensuring that in law it serves as a genuine 'boo-word' (see Archard, Chapter 5, p. 76).

However, postmodern interpretations of law would argue that law is heavily value laden (and historically contingent) in any event. Moreover, might it not be *more* damaging that populist morality finds expression in the extra-legal 'dialogic spaces' lying in the community domain? Is community scapegoating more or less intensive than that practised by the legislature, or by its courts, tribunals or local authorities? Irrespective of its scope and intensity, what about the lack of transparency (and procedural protections) in community settings? Was Simon right to prefer 'professionalisation' over 'proletarianisation' (participation or democracy)?

Communitarianism?

Communitarian scholars in North America tend to argue that a sound ethical base *will* emerge if there is space for 'extended, uncoerced, open conversation', which allows the Aristotelian idea of a consensus of '[p]hronesis, or practical knowledge' to emerge (Handler, 1988, pp. 1063–4). The French perspective developed by Ferry ('methodological communitarianism') baulks at adopting the cultural relativism embedded in the idea of phronesis, preferring a methodology which transcends context and permits universal ethical principles to be derived and applied (Ferry, 1994, pp. 299–300). One key to achieving this is addressing the structural 'limitations' of communication; in other words, cultivating the political institutions and cultural conventions of a genuinely pluralist and 'open society' (*ibid.*, pp. 302–3). But Ferry ends with an argument for incorporation of 'non- or irrational' views as well (*ibid.*, p. 306), perhaps raising doubts about whether communitarianism is able to resist the irrationalism of any incoming tide of community fear and loathing.

Handler's endorsement of dialogic community ideas is reassuring on these points, spelling out in great detail both the magnitude and complexity of the task of creating genuine dialogic spaces either within the bureaucracy (his main focus) or externally (as many continental theorists prefer). Notions of 'understanding *and* cooperation' are seen as central moral values (Handler, 1985, p. 1076, emphasis added). Relationships of trust must be built in place of mere mechanical contractual dealings (*ibid.*, p. 1078),[46] and community movements must be mobilized (particularly for dependent clients: *ibid.*, pp. 1108, 1112). Nor does Handler under-estimate the powerful contrary forces at work, including under-resourcing, power imbalances and unprofessional behaviour.

Certainly, the dialogic community, and the communitarian ethic it reflects (cf. MacIntyre, 1981), is a fragile alternative to legal liberalism and the associated legal-bureaucratic pattern characteristic of the postwar welfare state. Yet, as the Weberian model of law and administration crumbles and shrinks, it reinstates the reliance on the voluntarism, community support and private provision emblematic of nineteenth-century welfare and community organization.[47] Alternatives such as the dialogic community call for ever closer scrutiny – however fragile or contingent they may prove to be. As Fraser and Gordon (1994) point out, citizenship theory does not resonate in North America, accustomed as it is to a simple dichotomy between charity and 'contract'. In substance however, this reading of communitarianism equates with what is elsewhere termed 'neo-republican' citizenship.[48] Whatever its label, it may be an idea whose time has come.

Conclusion

What we have seen in this chapter is that there are at least two ways in which these citizenship rights and entitlements of children may be expressed: first in terms of protection against *negation* of those entitlements; and second, in terms of positively *securing* that access.[49]

The traditional late nineteenth-century welfare state sought to achieve its (limited) social policy objectives through a scheme of protective interventions (and associated institutional or other services), which were grounded in the moral innocence or perfectibility of children, and whose philosophic rationale was paternalism. It was an 'active' form of state mandate in child protection, but by the 1960s its force was spent, undone by the evidence of lack of success in achieving its idealistic gaols, and by clear indications of the heavy price paid in terms of incursions into the liberty of action of children and young people alike.

For a time, the 'rights movement' wrought a transformation of policy, splitting it into two arms. Protective intervention for its part reverted to a harms-based rationale during the late 1960s, a rationale more respectful of the due process (or civil citizenship) 'status' of children and families. Liberalism was revived. Services for children and families were altered too. The legacy of mainly 'institutional-based' services initially formed part of the passive citizenship of the 1940s welfare state. These too were reconceptualized as a more universal, non-stigmatizing expression of state obligations to assist and support citizens (children and their families) while they continued to live in the wider community, thus maximizing their potential for social participation. Briefly, the basic interests of children began to be recognized as an 'active' form of social citizenship rights.

Another way of expressing this is as a rebalancing of four main kinds of rights: 1) protective rights; 2) choice rights; 3) developmental rights; and 4) capacity rights (Sampford, 1986, pp. 32–3). What we have witnessed is that in place of policies grounded mainly in a 'protective' rationale, laws were rewritten to put more weight on negative (or 'choice') rights, while services became more reflective of 'positive' (or 'developmental') rights and the allied 'psychological' capacities required if citizens are meaningfully to exercise those rights. The latter are pivotal. This chapter has found classical liberalism wanting in its failure to recognize the 'connectedness' of human life.[50] Social citizenship rights are founded in social *relations*; it is not simply a question of the state providing a new entitlement (what the person *gets*) by making utilitarian policy calculations about what is or is not in the interests of the greatest good for the greatest number. It involves constructing *active* opportunities for the citizen to realize citizenship through what the person *does* (Davidson, 1997).

The question is whether law has a role to play in fostering environments where 'positive' or 'developmental' or more simply 'social' rights may flourish. Such rights rest in the application of the 'equality principle',[51] which is why their realization has been so dependent on the distributive arm of the welfare state over much of the course of the twentieth century. If they are not to be trumped by competing policy considerations, they must be expressed as 'ranking interests' in their own right; they cannot simply be derived from parental (and societal) interests in shaping future adults. Social reciprocity is the nub of this thesis: that citizen and state owe mutually responsible duties to each other; welfare is not simply a 'good' owed unconditionally to the citizen on preordained terms.

It is this reciprocity between citizens which builds the case for equivalent rights for adults in the aftermath of the transformation of the welfare state into the 'bargaining' or contractualist state spawned by contemporary values and trends, which seems likely to dominate at least the early stages of the twenty-first century. It is argued here that children of all ages are vulnerable to an erosion of their (few) public sector rights on two main fronts. They are vulnerable in a world tempted to demonize or otherwise scapegoat the young in response to societal insecurity stemming from economic change. And they are vulnerable to the rise of centrifugal moral forces associated with the rise of pluralism (often emblematic of that diverse body of scholarship travelling under the banner of 'postmodernism'). Plainly, privatization risks accentuating those dangers.

This threatens distributional justice for children. Diagnosis is comparatively easy. What is problematic is finding a convincing foundation for a new approach. The reciprocity characteristic of communitarian or genuinely contractual models make sense only for older (Gillick-competent: see Chapter 7) adolescents. For younger children the 'ethic of care and connection' is difficult to operationalize without compounding the impact of historical ideas such as 'good mothering'. Creative solutions may be needed if we are to bridge the public/private divide.

Some quite radical ideas give expression to this, such as New Zealand's use of 'family group conferences' to deal with the vast bulk of both delinquency and child protection matters, or North American 'sentencing circles'.[52] If properly designed, these certainly open the private spaces to incorporation of wider family and local community engagement.[53] However, they are vulnerable on another score: that minimum protections of justice and fairness may be jettisoned.[54] Less radical measures, such as tribunals or other 'popular' justice institutions may instead hold the key.[55]

Notes

1 LL.B(Hons), Dip. Crim. (Melb.), Ph.D. (Mon.), Professor of Law and former Head of Department, the University of Sydney. Part of this paper was written in 1996 while a Visiting Scholar, Social Policy Research Centre, University of New South Wales. Appreciation is expressed for the research assistance of Theresa Kelly LL.B(Hons) (Sheffield), Solicitor (England and Wales; NSW), and research funding provided by a grant from the NSW Law Foundation Legal Scholarship Scheme.
2 The looseness and ambiguity of language invites closer analysis to clarify meanings, but in cultural terms preservation of this ambiguity may be highly functional because it fosters dialogue essential to formation of common value positions.
3 Generally, I. Pinchbeck, and M. Hewitt, *Children in English Society,* London, Routledge and Kegan Paul, 1973.
4 Further, Marvell (1977) and Carson (1980).
5 Piper in this volume (ch. 3, pp. 39–49) argues that Britain was able to legislate against child employment and infanticide (baby farming) because risks such as undersocialization and creation of street children in competition with adults were focused on non-standard family units, and did not challenge the dominance of the prevailing family-centred system of religious morality. Delinquency measures too addressed aberrant families, who risked 'manufacture' of evil. While political and economic instability played some part in the latter, child protection initiatives had to await major recession and associated political instability.
6 See for example Murray (1985).
7 These developments have been charted by many writers, most relevantly for Australia and North America by Parker (1976), Platt (1977), Garlock (1979), and Gamble (1985), pp. 96–7.
8 This is most thoroughly reviewed in Seymour (1988). See also ALRC (1981), p. 12; Dingwall *et al.* (1984), p. 223.
9 Further, Horsburgh (1980).
10 King's 1981 argument went much too far in suggesting that welfare and justice were 'two sides of the same coin' and 'founded more on rhetoric than reality': King, (1981), p. 116. While it is true that both paradigms may be heavily infused with discretionary content, the same is true of public administration and its legal accountability under administrative law – yet no-one seriously argues that the executive and judicial branches of government can be equated here. It is also true (as argued here) that particular theories, principles, concepts and bodies of expertise will come into (and fall out of) fashion as public attitudes and values (or those of 'powerful groups': *ibid.*, p. 113) change, just as it is true that reliance on woolly concepts such as 'best interests of the child' facilitates this process (*ibid.*, pp. 129–30). But on the welfare/justice dichotomy King's proposi-

tion is that the more things change, the more they stay the same. Both
propositions cannot be equally valid. And whatever may be the position
in Britain, other countries have certainly witnessed real changes as justice
and welfare have ebbed and flowed: Naffine (1996).

11 Seymour (1985) provides a thorough review of these developments.

12 This is not to say that equal culpability necessarily dictates equal accountability under the criminal law (Richards, 1997, p. 87). Nor does it mean
that a moral calculus was displaced altogether by the reforms, even in
North America where this approach gained greatest sway (the converse of
Britain, where it gained hardly any currency at all). That child offender
legislation was dramatically reoriented in America in particular is not the
only dimension of this, of course. Even in countries where juvenile courts
retained either a middle position (Australia) or appeared to let it pass by
(Britain), it does not follow that public perceptions of juvenile offenders
were not significantly realigned with a 'needs' philosophy.

13 See, for example, Ramsland (1986) and Seymour (1988), ch. 1.

14 As evocatively expounded by Platt (1977).

15 Recent reviews include O'Connor (1997) and Naffine (1992).

16 The impact of the Convention, and the controversies it has provoked, are
nicely reviewed by Cohen and Miljeteig-Olssen (1991) and by
McGoldrick (1991).

17 See, for example, the discussions in Parker (1976), Ramsland (1986) and
Seymour (1988).

18 These debates within citizenship theory are well summarized by writers
such as Stewart (1995), Rees (1995) and Moon (1993).

19 Marshall's original essay is republished in Marshall (1973), pp. 67–127.
For an accessible contemporary discussion, see Kymlicka and Norman
(1994), pp. 352–81.

20 For an extended discussion of these ideas, see Harris (1987).

21 Simon (1986) pointed out that resort to concepts of property rather
impedes redistributive goals.

22 Her main argument is that positive (or welfare) entitlements to things
such as 'kindness', development of talents, 'involvement' or 'good feeling'
are imperfect obligations (not owed to every child like freedom from
sexual abuse) and not an incident of a *particular* relationship (such as carers
or teachers). Moreover, rights analysis is said to be of most political power
in correcting inappropriate repressive abuses of power, whereas children
are *legitimately* in need of dependent nurture (39–40). For a critique see
Coady (1992), pp. 49–50.

23 Further, Oldfield (1990), Leisink and Coenen (1993), pp. 5–6.

24 Thus Harris (1993b, p. 185) endorsed an integrative 'citizenship of entitlement' analysis in which the extension of civil and social rights are the
basis for participation by disadvantaged young people in the social and
economic life of the community.

25 For details of this saga, see Aldridge (1994) and Palmer (1996). The term
set by the minister was almost double the eight years envisaged by the
trial judge or the ten years contemplated by the Lord Chief Justice. Two
adverse rulings by the European Court of Human Rights ultimately led to
the restoration of some elements of due process and respect for the rule of

law with regard to release and recall procedures applied to children convicted of murder.

26 Finlayson (1994), pp. 9, 13–16.
27 This argument is elaborated and critiqued by writers such as Handler (1988), pp. 1043–4.
28 This argument is set out more fully in Carney (1991a).
29 These ideas are developed in Carney (1991b) and (1993).
30 See further, Carney (1994) and (1996). Conciliation or mediation of complex relational disputes appears to be superior to classical 'adjudication' of them (Carney, 1998).
31 Yeatman (1995) provides a good review of the elements and implications of contractualism.
32 See, for instance, the discussions by Hollingsworth (1996) and Prager (1992).
33 Weatherley (1994). Also Carney (1998).
34 Kosonen (1995), p. 820.
35 See Walby (1995) for an accessible treatment of this argument.
36 Clarke and Newman (1993), p. 47.
37 Latham (1996), p. 6.
38 This is elaborated elsewhere, see Carney (1996).
39 James and Jenks (1996) likewise muse over the implications of these trends in postmodern society, querying whether childhood is being reconstructed to amplify forms of state control (or Foucault's 'social policing'), while at the same time social insecurity may be leading people to invest ever more heavily in the myth of innocence, resolving the contradiction by demonizing extremes of childhood violence.
40 Simon argued that in choosing the 'professionalising' route ahead of its more democratic (or 'market' oriented) 'proletarianising' alternative, his solution at least had the attraction of '[P]romis[ing] to overcome some of the deficiencies of Weberian bureaucracy as an instrument of control and, by extending the reformer's own mode of life and work, to create valuable allies for her'. However

> [t]he disadvantages are, first, that if the strategy fails to inculcate the reformer's perspective, organisational autonomy may be used in ways that will frustrate her ends; and, second, that the expansion of professional status dilutes the exclusivity of the positions and perhaps the privileges of the reformer and her present allies.
> (Simon, 1983, p. 1262)

41 See, for example, Mnookin (1985).
42 Such a reconciliation of liberal and communitarian principles was foreshadowed by Freeman (1992), p. 54, n. 11.
43 A body of mainly US scholarship argues a more modest case, suggesting that substantive objectives of the law are appropriate, but should be recast to promote 'therapeutic' goals where this is not inconsistent with other values. See generally, D. Wexler (ed), *Therapeutic Jurisprudence: The Law as a Therapeutic Agent*, Durham NC: Carolina Academic Press, 1990; M.A. Levine, 'A therapeutic jurisprudence analysis of mandated reporting of child maltreatment by psychotherapists', *New York Law School Journal of*

Human Rights 10, 711, 1993; M. Perlin, 'What is therapeutic jurisprudence?', *New York Law School Journal of Human Rights* 10, 623, 1993.

44 Further, Handler (1988), p. 1047.
45 As was once done on the 'uncontrollable' child or 'exposure to moral danger' grounds for taking children into care, see Carney (1985).
46 Simon's decentralized professionalism may be a partial guarantor here. See Simon (1983), pp. 1195, 1199.
47 This is eloquently expounded in Finlayson (1994).
48 See, for example, Van Gunsteren (1994), p. 45.
49 Just over a decade ago Eekelaar spoke of a need to recognize 'basic interests' of children. These were said to encompass entitlements to 'general physical, emotional or intellectual care [which is] within the social capabilities of [the] immediate caregiver', see Eekelaar (1986), p. 170.
50 Further, Campbell (1992).
51 Dingwall and Eekelaar (1984), p. 106.
52 These models are reviewed and described by writers such as Morris and Maxwell (1995), La Prairie (1995) and O'Connor (1997), pp. 280–8.
53 Poorly designed programmes fail to engage the community, while however giving the appearance of doing so. For a recent critique of programmes allegedly sensitive to indigenous communities see, C. Cunneen, 'Community conferencing and the fiction of indigenous control', *Australian and New Zealand Journal of Criminology* 30, 292–311, 1997.
54 See for example Bargen (1995).
55 Such as continental multidisciplinary children's courts or Australia's experiment with tribunals to decide adult guardianship questions: see Carney and Tait (1997).

5   Can child abuse be defined?

David Archard

Why define child abuse?

No one would dispute that presently at the top or near the top of the agenda for the welfare of children is the detection and elimination of child abuse. Yet child abuse is a concept both lacking and in need of clear definition. Different and incompatible definitions of child abuse have been offered. There has been substantial and substantive disagreement about what the term means. When purportedly uncontentious general definitions have been provided they suffer from excessive vagueness and imprecision. The term's lack of clarity is consistent with its being widely and familiarly used. Indeed it may be the case that we are happier using the term while it remains ambiguous and unspecific. 'Maybe', concludes one expert reviewing writing on the subject, 'child abuse is too familiar a concept. We spend little time examining what we specifically mean by the term, preferring to spend our energies on the effects of abuse, methods of intervention, or other more direct and practical enterprises' (Gough, 1996, p. 993).

Nevertheless, a clear definition of child abuse is surely needed. 'We need to know what it is that we wish to prevent' (Gough and Murray, 1996, p. 203). The definition will fix the extent and seriousness of the problem, for how can we know how much there is of something without knowing precisely what it is that we are measuring. A definition will also help to determine the terms of research into the phenomenon, such as an inquiry into its causes and consequences. Finally, any definition will contribute to a specification of the criteria for action to deal with abuse, whether this action is legal, social or political.

The importance of definitional clarity derives most obviously from the fact that the term 'child abuse' has enormous evaluative force. It commands a moral response, one of unequivocal condemnation. What it designates is something that is plainly wrong. The term is thus what ordinary language philosophers used to characterize as a pejorative or 'boo-word'.[1] There is, moreover, a clear relationship between the descriptive scope of such a term and its condemnatory import. For we will remain comfortable in our use of the term only so long as we can be confident that what it represents out in the world merits being so strongly and immediately condemned. Consider, for example, the advertised claim that one in eight people was abused as a child.[2] If the claim were altered to one in three it would certainly be open to us to despair at the prevalence of so great an evil. Or we might quite simply judge that whatever is being described is so common an occurrence that it cannot, after all, be as bad as was once thought.

In this context the moral philosopher has an evident part to play: that of analysing the meaning of the term and evaluating the moral reasoning which supports the term's evaluative import. What sort of wrong is it that the term does or should isolate? And what grounds are there for thinking this to be as serious a wrong as agreed usage of the term would imply? There are two quite distinct worries about this sort of philosophical activity. The first is given admirable expression by David Gough in his review, already cited, of writing on child abuse:

> An examination of the meaning of the concept may be seen, at best, as an important but rather tedious and technical issue and, at worst, as an over-intellectual questioning of the meaning of abuse that implies that abuse does not really exist.
>
> (Gough, 1996, p. 13)

The second worry derives from a view that it is naïve to believe that a problem such as that of child abuse can be measured against univocal moral principles and remedied by the simple translation of agreed principles into effective social action. The philosopher's naïveté consists in both his or her understanding of society and the terms of social change, and a presumption of an achievable moral consensus.[3]

Defining harms to children

What follows is broadly philosophical in character. It does not indulge the conceit that real problems can be abolished simply by stipulating what a word shall or shall not mean; nor that social policy or political reform is merely applied ethics. However it does start from the belief that when we talk about child abuse we are, at a minimum, talking about something that is seriously bad and that should be reduced in its extent. It does not speculate on or make assumptions about how that reduction should be effected. Nevertheless it does suggest that the terms in which we talk about that problem are crucially important for the ways in which we might think about solving it – and that philosophical skills of analysis and evaluation might usefully inform the exercise of thinking about our use of the concept 'child abuse'. After all if the conclusion forced upon us is that the use of a distinct category of 'child abuse' is more of a hindrance than a help to the cause of improving children's lives, then the reasoning which led to that conclusion cannot be dismissed as mere idle speculation.

Let me start by stating that things do and can go badly for children in a variety of ways and for a number of reasons. Children may suffer a large range of harms. Some, such as illness, disease, genuine accidents, and disability, occur naturally. Others may be attributed to the actions of human beings or to the prevailing social circumstances. Some of the harms may be intentionally inflicted; others may be due to a failure to act in certain ways. No one further disputes that 'child abuse' does not exhaustively capture all of these harms. Child abuse is a special or significant kind of harm which befalls children, and it is normal to say that the harm is special or significant because it is particularly serious. It is fair to say – without prejudging issues that will be discussed later – that child abuse is significant harm to children and that its occurrence may be attributed to human agency. 'The two basic concepts underlying all definitions of abuse are harm and responsibility for that harm' (Gough, 1996, p. 996).

Here are two general definitions which try to capture this sense of the concept: 'Child abuse is a significant harm done or anticipated to a child as result of human action. That action may be intentional or reckless and inflicted by individuals, groups, agencies or the state' (Cooper, 1993, p. 1). 'Child abuse is the portion of harm to children that results from human action that is proscribed, proximate, and preventable' (Finkelhor and Korbin, 1988, p. 4).

These offerings are, in and because of their very generality, unavoidably vague. If we were to try to make them more precise what might we reasonably expect of the resultant definitions? Let me suggest that a clear working definition of child abuse should meet a number of requirements. These follow from what has already been said about the status of 'child abuse' as a 'boo-word'. First, the term should select some class of the harms which befall children according to a principle of selection which is evident and unambiguous. The term should be employable in such a way that we can readily say of some set of circumstances that it is bad for the children involved but that it is not abuse or not yet abuse. Second, the term should define a class of harms which are uniform in some important or salient respect. Instances of abuse should display a commonality of character. We need not specify necessary and sufficient conditions for the application of the concept, but there ought at least to be family resemblances between whatever is defined by it. If that requirement cannot be met, then there is no reason why we cannot speak just in general terms of harm to children's interests, and think of a broad range of actions and conditions which occasion varying degrees of such harm.

Non-contentiousness

The third requirement of a definition of 'child abuse' is that its constitutive terms should not be contentious. The concept cannot have clear evaluative connotations if it is defined in ways that are not evaluatively clear to everyone. There is also a now familiar background principle of law- and policy-making in a liberal society which demands that a government be officially neutral with regard to conceptions of the good. A state should not invoke, in justification of any of its measures, moral understandings, values or precepts that are disputed by some within its jurisdiction. A definition of child abuse should not be non-neutral, as the philosopher Gerald Dworkin defines it, where a non-neutral principle is one whose 'application to particular cases is a matter of controversy for the parties whose conduct is supposed to be regulated by the principle in question' (Dworkin, 1974, p. 492).

It should be evident that the scope of neutrality must be restricted to reasonable views. A definition of child abuse cannot, for instance, be neutral with regard to the paedophiliac view that sexual activity between an adult and a young child need not be to the detriment of the latter and may indeed be to his or her benefit. It is reasonable to believe that the objections of paedophiles to principles which prohibit their own activity should be discounted. This is not to say that paedophiles have not mounted and do not try to mount a reasoned defence of their own sexual preferences (O'Carroll, 1980; Gough, 1981; Califia, 1981). Such a defence does not, explicitly, state that the wishes of children should be ignored. But in so far as it does suggest that children may welcome and encourage sexual encounters with adults, its portrayal of children as complicit in their own abuse amounts to a false and self-serving rationalization. Which is to say that paedophilia can only be defended if the interests, needs and wishes of other parties, namely children, are themselves discounted. In this sense, a defence of paedophilia cannot be 'reasonable'.

Definitions of abuse should try to avoid key terms which display an 'open texture'.[4] This is when a word's precise definition and application are open to reasonable disagreement between people who nevertheless can agree that they are using the same word. Consider, for instance, how one should understand the scope of a principle which invokes a standard of the 'proper', 'normal' or 'adequate' care of a child. What these terms might actually imply in concrete terms is open to considerable variation between cultures, ages and communities. The resultant problem is simply that their precise meaning can only be the subject of discretionary interpretation by whoever is in a position to apply the principles in question.

The fourth requirement of a category of 'child abuse' is that its avoidance or prevention should not impose impossible or unreasonable demands on those charged with the responsibility of caring for a child. This requirement follows from the fact that, as already noted, abuse is a harm to children which may be attributed to human agency. It follows from this fact in conjunction with the familiar principle that responsibility or liability for the occasioning of some wrong is only fairly ascribed if the wrong could have been avoided. Abuse is avoidable and we should be in a position to contrast those who do not abuse their children with those who need not but do abuse their children.

It is, of course, vital that we do not prejudge the question of the source of the avoidable human action. The two general definitions of abuse quoted above are both careful not to do so. Note that the first speaks of action by 'individuals, groups, agencies or the state' and that the second speaks only of 'human action'. In the wake of the modern discovery of child abuse came a realization that it ought to be possible, and on occasion essential, to speak of 'collective abuse'; that is the abuse of children the responsibility for which was attributable to social, political or economic institutions, practices or arrangements. It should not, in other words, be assumed that the abuse of a child can only be maltreatment at the hands of an individual adult such as a parent or carer. Children can, it is argued, be abused when their social and economic circumstances are such that their interests are seriously damaged. Or, most poignantly, when the welfare system designed to protect them from individual abuse only subjects them to further significant harms.

Whilst it may not be improper to speak of 'collective abuse' – and this is a subject to which I will return – it is proper that such abuse, if it is agreed to exist, should be avoidable. This does not mean that any one individual is able to prevent it. It is rather that the institutional arrangements could be changed in such a way that the abuse no longer occurred. If children suffer serious illness and death due to poor social conditions which society could (and, we judge, should) improve then this would be collective abuse.[5] That the children suffer the same degree of ill-health due to the spread of a contagious illness that could neither have been foreseen nor prevented is not abuse.

There are other requirements of a concept of child abuse which are less important for present purposes but which may be summarized briefly at this point. The concept should be sufficiently flexible to accommodate the discovery of new forms of what are undoubtedly abusive behaviours towards children. Nothing in the definition should rule this out. So, for instance, it should be possible to characterize as abuse Munchausen syndrome by proxy, a phenomenon which is at present of concern to many people engaged in preventing child abuse. A definition also should not rule out (any more than it should automatically rule in) the organized ritual abuse of children.

Another requirement is that the definition of child abuse should not be of a kind which settles in advance the question of how abuse is to be explained. The term may well cover a variety of conditions and actions, each of which has its own distinctive set of causes. It need not be the case that all forms of child abuse have a single root cause. Of course, as the second requirement of an adequate definition stipulated, instances of child abuse should be uniform in some important or salient respect. But the question of what child abuse *is*, what makes each and every instance of abuse fall under the same general concept, should be kept separate from the issue of how each of these various instances is to be causally explained. So, for instance, it may be plausible to think that poverty is or can be an important part of the explanation for the neglect of children. It is not plausible to think that the sexual abuse of children also and as clearly correlates with poverty.

Orthodox and persuasive definitions

It may well be that there is no single overarching definition of child abuse which meets these suggested requirements. It may be that at most a satisfactory concept of child abuse will comprise a list of different possible particular kinds of abuse. However, let me acknowledge that a great deal of published material – taking the form of generally consulted studies of child abuse and official government or international policy guidelines – operates with what I will call the *orthodox narrow definition of child abuse*. Particular formulations of this definition may differ in degree but all conform to a similar pattern. It is an umbrella definition in that a number of kinds of abuse come under it. They come under it in so far as they all display the general characteristics of abuse identified in the overarching definitions quoted earlier (Cooper, 1993, p. 1; Finkelhor and Korbin, 1988, p. 4).

The orthodox definition considers child abuse to have four subcategories: physical abuse, physical neglect, sexual abuse and emotional abuse. Let me give an example of a definition of each subcategory. Physical abuse is 'violence and other non accidental, prohibited human actions that inflict pain on a child and are capable of causing injury or permanent impairment to development or functioning' (Finkelhor and Korbin, 1988, p. 8). Physical neglect is the 'persistent or severe neglect of a child (for example, by exposure to any kinds of danger, including cold and starvation) which results in serious impairment of the child's health or development, including non-organic failure to thrive' (Department of Health and Social Services, 1991a). Sexual abuse is 'the involvement of dependent, developmentally immature children and adolescents in sexual activities that they do not fully comprehend, are unable to give informed consent to, and that violate the social taboos of family roles' (Schechter and Roberge, 1976, p. 129). Emotional abuse or psychological maltreatment is 'a concerted attack on a child's development of self and social competence, a *pattern* of psychically destructive behavior, and it takes five forms: *Rejecting...Isolating...Terrorizing...Ignoring...Corrupting*' (Garbarino *et al.*, 1986, p. 8). Some versions of the orthodox definition have included a further category of 'grave concern'. But this was designed to pick out children at serious risk of abuse or suspected of suffering abuse rather than itself designating a type of abuse.

The definition instanced above is orthodox in that it figures in official documents, and narrow in so far as it understands child abuse to be limited to a constrained group of specific, serious harms. However, ever since child abuse was first discovered the term has been subject to 'persuasive definition'. This philosophical term was coined by Charles L. Stevenson in 1938:

> A 'persuasive' definition is one which gives a new conceptual meaning to a familiar word without substantially changing its emotive meaning, and which is used with the conscious or unconscious purpose of changing, by this means, the direction of people's interests.
>
> (Stevenson, 1938, p. 331)

So someone offering a persuasive definition of child abuse may seek to persuade people that something, not previously covered by the term, is child abuse and should be viewed with the same disapproval that attaches to all other instances of child abuse. The scope of the 'boo-word' is extended even whilst its capacity to evoke a 'boo' is retained. Indeed that is the point of persuasive definition.

As philosophers have noted, terms such as 'real', 'genuine' or 'true' often accompany persuasive definitions. For instance, anti-abortionists frequently remark that abortion is the real or true child abuse that occurs in our society. The purpose of such persuasive definition is to get us to recognize that any horror felt at what we currently acknowledge to be abuse should be felt – more strongly and with even more reason to be felt – at what the definition is extended to include. Consider – as an example of broadening the scope of the term without diluting its evaluative import – David Gil's influential definition of child abuse as 'inflicted gaps or deficits between circumstances of living which would facilitate the optimal development of children to which they would be entitled and their actual circumstances, irrespective of the sources or agents of the deficit' (Gil, 1975, pp. 346–7). If this definition were accepted and adopted then all those children living in or on the margins of poverty in our society would be properly described as abused. And their condition would have to be regarded with the same horrified disapproval that accompanies any other instance of abuse.

Persuasive definition is not of itself illicit, though philosophers, like everyone else, view with suspicion any attempt to win a case or make a point simply by changing the meaning of words. Any change in the definition of a term needs to be supported by independent argument and evidence. Moreover there is a well-grounded presumption that the definition of a term is properly given, at least in the first instance, by established or customary usage.

The problems of fixing meanings

There are at least two reasons why child abuse has been subject to persuasive definition and why it is difficult to retain a fixed, constrained understanding of the term. The first is that child abuse is a *modern discovery*. There are three moments in this discovery: agitation around the issue of child cruelty by emergent welfare organizations at the end of the nineteenth century (see Chapter 3); the disclosure and labelling of the 'battered child syndrome' in 1962; and the growing awareness from the 1970s onward of the extent of child sexual abuse. To say that child abuse is a modern discovery is not to say that before this century children were not subjected to the same forms of cruel and neglectful behaviour as now. It is to say that a term or concept has come into accepted usage, by means of which behaviours and states of affairs – both past and present – can now and for the very first time be labelled and described.

The relevant effects of the concept's modernity are twofold. First, there is a lack of confidence in the concept's meaning which might otherwise have come from long-established usage. A term without clear provenance is one whose definition is easier to manipulate and change. Second, the newness of the concept reinforces its status as a 'human kind' concept. This is contrasted with a 'natural kind' concept, one which represents how nature really is and has always been, how it is 'carved at the joints'. A human kind concept is artificial in the sense both that it represents what is the artifice of human kind and that it is itself the construction of human language and thought. It is thus often said that the idea of 'child abuse' is the product of social construction (Gelles, 1975; Pfohl, 1977). Anything which has been constructed can, of course, be re-constructed, extended and altered.

The second reason why the definition of child abuse has been difficult to fix is that, from the beginning, there have been a variety of interested groups seeking to supply the definitive account of the phenomenon. Each has sought to do so in so far as a definition of child abuse will imply a causal explanation, an aetiology of the phenomenon, in the light of which that group, perhaps alone, can claim to have the resources to understand and act. Thus whereas the early voluntary agencies such as the NSPCC and Barnardos sought to give themselves an officially sanctioned role in the detection and remedying of child cruelty (Behlmer, 1982), it was paediatricians who offered a medicalized account of the battered child in 1962 (Kempe, 1962).

Child 'cruelty' was disclosed at the turn of this century. Child 'abuse' proper was discovered in the early 1960s. Since this latter date the concept has been subject to continuous adaptation. It has, as Ian Hacking the philosopher and historian of ideas has noted, 'not been fixed during the quarter century of its existence. Malleable and expansionist, it has gobbled up more and more kinds of bad acts' (Hacking, 1988, p. 54). '[N]o one had any glimmering, in 1960, of what was going to count as child abuse in 1990' (Hacking, 1991, p. 257). The claim so far is that the circumstances of the concept's origin and subsequent development – its comparative newness and the fact that a number of different groups have sought to supply a definitive account of it – have given it an understandable malleability. There are still further reasons why it may be difficult to fix the meaning and scope of the term. I will state what I take these to be and then, given everything that has been said, I will try to say something about the future for a concept of 'child abuse' which meets the definitional requirements listed earlier.

It was stated that the core understanding of child abuse is that it is significant harm to children whose occurrence may be attributed to human agency. The reasons for fearing that it may be very hard to fix the meaning of 'child abuse' have to do with the difficulties of specifying the agreed meanings of the constitutive terms of this understanding – namely, 'significant harm' and 'human agency'. There are three main difficulties. The first concerns 'human agency'. Earlier it was acknowledged that it may be proper to speak of 'collective abuse' and that definitions of abuse are often carefully formulated so as not to prejudge the nature of the agency which is held responsible for the harms to children. All that is required is that the social, economic or political practices, institutions and arrangements held accountable for the ills that befall children should be alterable. It then seems plausible to argue as follows. A society which conscripts its young children into active armed service or which denies them the food, shelter, education and health care which it reasonably could provide them with is abusing them. Where there is no good morally relevant difference between harms that are individual in origin and those that are collectively caused, any definition which seeks to specify a certain kind of harm should not exclude the possibility of these having their source in a collective agency.

However the possibility of attributing agency – of a kind which allows us to speak of responsibility or liability for the causing of harm – to social or collective entities is contested. Indeed, a familiar and long-standing debate within social and political philosophy concerns the propriety of ascriptions of moral agency to anything other than individuated human beings. Note that the question is not whether significant harms befall children because they live under certain kinds of social and political arrangements. That can be conceded. The question is rather whether they are *wronged* by so living, where the accusation of wrongdoing presupposes responsibility and the responsibility is laid at the door of the set of arrangements. It does not help to try and offer a reduction of collective responsibility. That is to attempt to translate any story of 'collective' abuse into a story which refers only to the actions of individuals. This is not useful because the very possibility of such a successful translation is just what is at stake in the dispute between a 'collectivist' and an 'individualist'.

Turning to the second constitutive term of child abuse there are two reasons to think that it is difficult to fix the meaning of what shall count as 'significant' or 'serious' harm to a child. The first is the straightforward evidence of considerable historical and cultural variance in this matter. In support of his master claim that society prior to the modern period lacked a concept of childhood Philippe Ariès cites the fact that in earlier periods forms of behaviour towards children which we would now deem grossly inappropriate were tolerated, indeed encouraged. An example would be the participation of children in sexually explicit conduct.[6] The evidence of cultural variance is equally striking.[7] Consider the following. In a sub-Saharan African tribal society a parent scarifies the face and body of her child. In another the young boys are fellated by elders as part of the former's initiation ceremony. Infants are genitally stimulated to induce relaxation and sleep. Young children are set to work in the fields alongside adults. There are societies whose young girls are subjected to clitoridectomy and infibulation. In China young girls had their feet bound. Non-Western cultures view some of our child-rearing practices as unnecessarily cruel, for instance compelling children to eat according to strict regimen or leaving them to sleep alone and apart from their parents.

There are two sources of societal or cultural variation, one of which is more troubling than the other. The less worrying source of variation is that one and the same instance of behaviour towards a child may be invested with a different significance or meaning in different cultures. Thus deliberate scarifying is a form of beautification and not, as it would be in another context, mutilation. Again, the fellating of adolescents is not for the sexual gratification of the adults, but is rather seen in terms of an initiation into the group and the transmission of certain powers across generations.

The second source of variance, however, arises because of deepseated disagreements about what is proper and acceptable treatment of children. In this instance the disagreements cannot be explained away in terms of the different significance of the same behaviour in various contexts. Rather what one culture regards as permissible or appropriate another finds unacceptable. The belief that there is a single standard of morally acceptable behaviour towards children, and that this standard is to be found operating in our own society, may rest upon ethnocentric assumptions of cultural superiority. However a toleration of all standards, where these do differ significantly, commits the sin of moral relativism (see Chapter 6). An understanding of child abuse which avoids appeal to any contested norm of appropriate behaviour is most likely to be emptied of substantive content. Or it will presuppose so low a minimally acceptable level of conduct as to exclude only the very worst kinds of harm. By contrast, a definition of child abuse which has substance will probably fall foul of the requirement that it be specified in neutral ways.

A splendid illumination of the difficulties faced in this context can be found in the deliberations behind the drafting of the agreed terms of the United Nations Convention on the Rights of the Child. The existence of international organizations dedicated to the promotion of children's welfare world-wide (such as, most notably, UNICEF) and the codification of the fundamental rights of children to whose protection and promotion all governments should be devoted (such as, most obviously, the UN Convention) has done much to draw attention to the status and well-being of children globally. However, any agreement across very different political, religious, moral and cultural identities and traditions about how, even at a minimum, children should be treated has been secured only by deliberate ambiguity of language or resort to the lowest common denominator.[8]

The third reason it is difficult to fix the definition of child abuse is that any plausible definition of abuse must invoke a benchmark or baseline of a child's normal health and development. This is because an entity can be harmed not merely in being positively damaged but, negatively, in falling below what would otherwise be its normal or expected state. Consider this formulation from the English Children Act: 'Where the question of whether harm suffered by a child is significant turns on the child's health or development, his health or development shall be compared with that which could reasonably be expected of a similar child' (Children Act 1989, Section 4, (31)(10)).

There may, in similar terms, be reference to the normal standard of care. Whatever terms are used – 'reasonable', 'expected', 'acceptable', 'normal', 'adequate' or 'proper' – they specify a baseline. And any baseline may be set at a higher or lower level. In the Children Act the baseline is set by reference to what might be 'expected of a similar child'. But of course it is then reasonable to ask, 'similar in what respects?' Are these specified in terms of age, class background, national origin, or what? To each of these possibilities, and others, there corresponds a higher or lower baseline.

In general there are at least three different levels at which a baseline of normal development and health might be set. For each there is a correspondingly different understanding of what counts as a departure from the norm, and thus what counts as significant harm, and thus what counts as abuse. The lowest is one set in terms of minimum or basic needs. It will specify the food, shelter, health care, and parental care which a child needs simply in order to survive. Such a level may seem implausibly low. It will not, for instance, allow us to characterize as abusive any parental behaviour which only just meets the basic needs of a child, but is otherwise cold and uncaring by the standards operating elsewhere in the same society.

The second level at which the baseline of normality may be set is according to the standards of a particular community. 'According to this approach behaviour which falls below the community norm and also results in specifiable harm would be abusive or neglectful. It is this standard which is employed in cases charging negligence' (Abrams, 1979, p. 157). At this level the baseline specifies what a society, by its own lights, deems to be good enough for its children. The distinction between satisfying universal basic needs and meeting the terms of what is minimally acceptable within a society, that between the first and second levels, parallels the distinction between absolute and relative poverty. In both cases what counts as falling below the line will vary across societies and over time. Using such a standard allows us to be sensitive to the prevailing norms within a community and to differences between communities. However, it does present problems. What one society deems good enough care for its children may be viewed as grossly unacceptable by another. Moreover it seems counterintuitive to describe as abusive any behaviour which more than meets the basic needs of a child, but which falls short of the very high standards which happen to be set in some particular society but no other.

The highest level of the baseline is one set in terms of the best possible upbringing. David Gil's definition of abuse, quoted earlier, spoke of it as any gap between the actual circumstances of a child and those 'which would facilitate [its] optimal development'. Such an optimizing benchmark seems implausible. Abuse is surely much more than a failure simply to do the best that one can for a child. Any such failure will not necessarily, indeed will rarely, result in the significant avoidable harm to a child which we think of as abuse. If it is pointed out that Gil talks of the optimal development to which children would be 'entitled', the obvious reply is that the extent of any such entitlements are open to serious, and probably irresolvable, disagreement. Or that such disagreement can be resolved only by specifying the entitlements either in terms of a basic minimum set of needs or in terms of community norms. In which case the third level collapses into the first or second.

These are then three grounds for thinking it difficult to fix a definition of child abuse which meets the stipulation that such a definition is non-contentious and yet picks out an interesting, salient class of significant harms to children which can reasonably be avoided. These grounds compound the pressures persuasively to define and simply to extend or alter the concept of child abuse. Does then the concept of child abuse have a viable and socially valuable future? What role, if any, should it play within a moral agenda for children's welfare? How, in the final analysis, ought we to understand and define child abuse? Answering these sorts of questions is not possible here. Moreover attempting to do so, even briefly, might run the risk of confirming those criticisms of philosophical inquiry which were cited at the outset of this chapter. These were that such inquiry linguistically legislates the problem of abuse out of existence. And that it is detached from a serious examination of, and thereby badly misunderstands, the conditions of possibility of social change.

Conclusion

Rather than run those risks here I will conclude by outlining, in a very schematic way, three ways in which talk about the welfare of children, in so far as it does or does not involve use of a concept of child abuse, might develop. The first would be settled and agreed usage of the orthodox narrow definition of child abuse with further attempts to broaden the term, such as might be entailed by persuasive definitions, being defeated. The second would be what Hacking called the 'malleable' and 'expansionist' development of the term as it 'gobbles up more and more kinds of bad act'. The third would involve the concept of child abuse ceasing to have any further use. Instead there would simply be talk of a range of harms that may befall children through the action and inaction of human agency. Rather than singling out any particular class of such harms as 'abuse' the different degrees of harmfulness involved in all such harmful behaviours would be categorized.

The conditions under which the concept of child abuse was born and those under which it must continue to flourish may be such as to make it impossible to hope that it can have a clear fixed definition which meets the requirements listed earlier. Yet definitional expansionism can reduce the effectiveness – in discourses of moral criticism – of a 'boo-' (and also a 'hurrah-') word. A good parallel example is provided by the expansionist use of the language of rights. As L. Sumner notes there has been an 'escalation of rights rhetoric' as more and more rights have been claimed by more and more groups in respect of more and more things. He comments:

Inflation devalues a currency by eroding its purchasing power. The proliferation of rights claims has devalued rights by eroding their argumentative power....As a concept is stretched further and further beyond its proper domain it is also emptied of more and more of its distinctive content. Thus the increasing versatility of rights has been purchased at the cost of their increasing vacuity.

(Sumner, 1987, p. 15)

We might similarly say that the increasing versatility of the concept of child abuse – its ability to pick out more and more types of wrong done to children – has only been purchased at the cost of its increasing vacuity, its lack of any distinctive content possessing clear evaluative connotations. On the other hand, allowing the concept of child abuse to fall into desuetude might risk a failure to notice a distinctive class of harms to which children are subject and which deserve our particular attention. Perhaps we do need reminding that some things which are done or happen to children are beyond the pale and must come top of the agenda for children's welfare. Neglecting what is properly isolated as the 'abuse of children' and as a result resorting to general talk only of 'harms' to them might mean – to use a horribly appropriate metaphor – throwing the baby out with the bathwater.

Notes

1 Cranston (1953), p. 16, for instance, picks out 'liberty' as a 'hurrah-word' and 'license', by contrast, as a 'boo-word'.
2 'One in every eight people who walk past this poster was abused as a child', NSPCC hoarding advertisement, 'A cry for the child', 1996.
3 For a critique along these sorts of lines, see King (1997), especially ch.1.
4 The phrase is H.L.A. Hart's describing the necessarily indeterminate character of legal language (Hart, 1961, p. 124ff.).
5 This claim need involve no naïve view of society as a self-reforming agent (of the sort subject to criticism for its sociological naïveté). It requires only that there be in place political procedures for introducing and implementing policy measures with the purpose of, and effective in, ameliorating the poor social conditions in question.
6 'One of the unwritten laws of contemporary morality, the strictest and best respected of all, requires adults to avoid any reference, above all any humorous reference, to sexual matters. This notion was entirely foreign to the society of old.' Ariès instances Heroard's diary, which records the upbringing of the young Louis XIII, and notes that a modern reader of this diary 'is astonished by the liberties which people took with children, by the coarseness of the jokes they made, and by the indecency of gestures made in public which shocked nobody and were regarded as perfectly natural' (Ariès, 1962, p. 100).

7 A very useful text here is Korbin (1981).

8 An example within the UN Convention in the context of measures to promote children's health is the deliberate decision to avoid any specific mention of female circumcision and, instead, speak only of 'traditional practices'. A study of the UN Convention comments on this, 'It is one of the most important examples of how the cultural diversity of the United Nations forced a compromise that, rather than making advances in the area of children's rights, actually resulted in the adoption of very weak norms' (LeBlanc, 1995, p. 89).

6 Is male circumcision morally defensible?

Ilan Katz

There was excitement in the crowd, and I shuddered slightly, knowing that the ritual was about to begin....The old man would use his assegai to change us from boys to men with a single blow....Before I knew it, the old man was kneeling in front of me....His hands moved so fast they seemed to be controlled by an outworldly force. Without a word he took my foreskin, pulled it forward, and then, in a single motion, brought down his assegai. I felt as if fire was shooting through my veins; the pain was so intense that I buried my chin in my chest. Many seconds seemed to pass before I remembered the cry, and then I recovered and called out, 'Ndiyindonda' (I am a man)....I felt ashamed that the other boys seemed much stronger and firmer than I had....A boy may cry; a man conceals his pain.

(Mandela, 1994, pp. 25–6)

Female circumcision...is a cultural tradition which needed to be challenged. There is now a body of people from both the Muslim and Jewish religions who are beginning to doubt the efficacy of male circumcision....There is also discrepancy as to the history of the act. For some, it has a religious validity; for others, it separates the cultures and therefore should be maintained. For people like myself who do not have those traditions to consider, it appears barbaric and abusive. I defy anyone who has witnessed either of these two acts to still maintain that it is pain-free and harmless.

(Jackson, 1996, pp. 16–17)

Why is circumcision a moral issue?

On the face of it, circumcision is not a moral issue at all. It is a very widespread phenomenon which is practised by a large proportion of the world's cultures. Although there are no figures, it is clear that virtually every adult male Muslim, African and Jew, along with many others, has been circumcised. In the earlier part of this century most male children in the UK and USA were circumcised. Surely such a widely prevalent practice cannot be morally wrong? In general male circumcision is seen as a cultural practice which is fairly harmless and of little consequence for the moral debate around children. Yet there are rumblings of discontent coming from various quarters.

Probably the most significant source of tension is the question of female circumcision or female genital mutilation (FGM), which is seen to be a major moral issue, being subject to a UN resolution and several international conferences, and which is forbidden by law in the UK. The unspoken question is, of course, why are these two forms of circumcision or genital mutilation treated so differently – are the differences merely quantitative or are there qualitative differences between them? The similarities and differences between male and female circumcision will be further discussed below.

The second rumble has come from the occasional media foray into the subject, especially the programme *It's a Boy!* shown in the UK on Channel 4 in 1995, which examined the problem of male circumcision. This was a powerful programme which caused much debate in the Jewish community, mainly because the director was a Jewish man and the programme was very well made. The programme included input from 'defenders' of circumcision, but they tended to come across as inarticulate and patronizing, rather than as really addressing the issue. Nevertheless, the subject is, in the main, conspicuous by its absence. An Internet search revealed thirty-one articles on circumcision, but only two on male circumcision, both relating to medical considerations.

This chapter will argue that the logic of child protection[1] lies with Jackson rather than Mandela, and that this logic, which underpins professional thinking about children, must see circumcision as abusive and morally wrong. This chapter will also argue, however, that this conclusion is dependent on a system of thought and a reasoning which is not shared by minority communities and that, despite the heavy emphasis placed on culturally sensitive and anti-racist practice, the rationale of child protection cannot deal with rites such as circumcision. I will argue that from a different standpoint it may be morally wrong and indeed abusive for a Jewish child *not* to be circumcised. Because child protection and cultural practices come from different moral universes, I will conclude that there can be no real argument between them, and that ultimately the issue of which of them is morally right is undecidable.

This chapter is written from the point of view of a male secular[2]

Jew. Like the overwhelming majority of secular Jews, I was quite proud to circumcise my sons, and saw their circumcision as a slightly risky but inevitable duty which needed to be undertaken if they were to take their places in the community. Like most Jews I did not see it as a moral issue, and only the recent debates have made me re-evaluate my attitude towards circumcision. Paradoxically, this has led me to re-evaluate my own views of child protection practice and cultural sensitivity. In this article I will focus on the Jewish experience of circumcision. In other cultures there are some similar arguments and dynamics in force, but some of the issues are different. In particular, Judaism is probably unique in that circumcision takes place at a very early age (eight days) so the possibility of obtaining the child's own perceptions does not exist. Circumcision also has a particular place in the culture which may or may not be similar to that of other cultures. The quote above from Nelson Mandela is interesting in that it is a first-person account of circumcision, which of course would not be available from a Jewish point of view, but which illustrates how different thinking can be from the Western humanist perspective.

It must be emphasized that for religious Jews there is no moral debate at all. Circumcision has been commanded by God as part of his covenant with the Jewish people, and for a religious Jew it is a *Mitzvah* – a holy duty as well as a source of pleasure in fulfilling an important commandment. From this standpoint, those who oppose circumcision (at least by Jews) are opposing the word of God, and there is no point in debating with them. Additionally, for religious Jews, abandoning circumcision would amount to abandoning Judaism as a culture, and therefore would have significance beyond the individuals who are not circumcised. Circumcision is not only a religious rite, but a defining feature of the Jewish ethnic group. For religious Jews, therefore, the moral issue is not about injuring children but about observing the will of God. Not to circumcise a male child is therefore wrong because it:

- contravenes the *halachah* (Jewish law)
- denies the child the blessing of full Jewishness
- defies the covenant between God and the Jewish people.

Secular Jews do not see circumcision as a divine commandment. For most secular Jews, however, the continuation of the Jewish culture is important, and requires some personal effort. This may involve adherence to dietary and Sabbath laws, attendance at synagogue or celebrating major festivals. Even Jews who perform none of these religious duties regard circumcision as a defining characteristic of their ethnic identity, and the practice is almost universal. Hoffman says: 'throughout time...the rite of circumcision has steadfastly remained the single most obvious boundary issue, marking the limits beyond which Jews felt that they could not go without at the same time leaving Judaism' (Hoffman, 1996, p. 12).

From this point of view, a decision not to circumcise a child has risks and consequences. The risk for the individual child is that not being circumcised will lead to exclusion from his community, and will rob him of the possibility of being fully Jewish. More importantly, for both religious and secular Jews, there would be consequences for the community as a whole, which is seen as being threatened in a fundamental way by the denial of this practice. On the other hand, some secular Jews are concerned about the risks to their children and about the pain of the rite. Many, especially women, are concerned about the androcentric symbolism which lies at the core of the rite. It is for secular Jews that circumcision becomes a moral issue in the sense discussed here.

There are two reasons why male circumcision can be seen as morally wrong. The most obvious is that circumcision involves physically injuring a child. The second reason is that male circumcision, despite the fact that it is males who are being injured, is a decidedly patriarchal practice. In all cultures in which male circumcision is practised, it symbolizes a rite of passage for males into the community, either as the beginning of adulthood or as a member of the community itself. The implication is that only men can be true members of the community. In the Jewish *Brith Milah* (circumcision ceremony), women are excluded altogether. Historically, circumcision was associated with male blood, which was seen as 'purifying', in contrast with the 'impure' menstrual blood of women (Hoffman, 1996).

Thus circumcision transgresses two fundamental moral values which are central to the humanist liberalism which underpins Western professionalism – the rights of children to physical integrity and the rights of women to equality. Importantly, these values are accepted as being universal and not culturally bound, and are enshrined in UN resolutions and charters.

Cultural sensitivity

Cultural sensitivity is addressed in the literature as part of anti-oppressive, anti-racist and multicultural models. It is usually seen as a subcategory of anti-racism, which views cultural sensitivity within the wider contexts of the power differentials between members of minority ethnic communities and white people. The literature almost invariably addresses situations in which the minority members are the service users, and professionals carrying out statutory child protection functions are white, thus increasing the differences in power and resources.

Unfortunately, 'cultural sensitivity', (along with 'empowerment', 'partnership', etc.) is one of those concepts which, although universally and uncritically adopted by the helping professions,[3] is riven with moral contradictions, making it virtually impossible to incorporate it coherently into practice. Multiculturalism was strongly advocated by progressive educationalists in the 1970s and early 1980s, and had an important influence on professional thinking, especially in social work. It was, however, superseded by anti-racism because it had two fundamental weaknesses:

- It failed to address the issues of racism and colonialism in its analysis, and conceived of cultural differences simply as different ways of viewing the world. It therefore ignored how power relationships, rather than 'misunderstandings' were central to race relations (see Dutt and Phillips, 1996).
- It had a tendency to perpetuate the power of (usually male) elites who defined the norms within minority cultures so that the needs of less powerful or marginalized members of minority communities were ignored (Frosh, Chapter 12, this volume).

Nevertheless, the 'modernist anti-racist' attack on multiculturalism allowed most of its tenets to be incorporated into a larger anti-racist agenda. Cultural sensitivity has remained part of the anti-oppressive paradigm, and is still subject to many conceptual difficulties.

First, culturally sensitive practice assumes that there are uncontested norms in each culture which are easily used as parameters or benchmarks by which the actions of individual members of the group can be measured. 'Cultures' are defined (if at all) in their structuralist mode – i.e. as a set of practices or behaviours which are accepted by a particular ethnic group. The deficiencies of this notion have been extensively written about (Rattansi, 1992), but have not entered legal and social work decisions concerning children's welfare (Katz, 1996a).

Another problem is that cultural sensitivity (or cultural relativity) is always selective or 'relatively relative'. Certain customs are deemed to be appropriate for minority cultures to practice, while some practices are seen as universal. Often it is the superficial manifestations of a culture, such as food, dress, music, etc., which are viewed with sympathy and displayed on classroom walls. The values by which individuals live do not generally attract as much attention or the support of professionals, especially when they contradict strongly held tenets of anti-racist orthodoxy (Cohen, 1992).

Cultural sensitivity takes a deficiency stance towards the 'other'. Despite constant exhortations in the literature to adopt a 'difference' rather than a 'deficiency' model of culture (e.g. Korbin, 1993; Keats, 1997), liberal humanist cultural values are inevitably the yardstick by which minorities are measured. If necessary, cultural relativity accepts that our value systems should be relaxed to accommodate others whose standards are different. Crucially, however, Western liberal values are not themselves seen as amenable to change or challenge by other cultural beliefs and practices. For example, in many Muslim communities in the UK it is viewed as abusive of parents *not* to send their children to a religious school, but not at all abusive to physically chastise a child who refuses to go to school (Katz, 1996b). It is quite likely that physical chastisement will result in the intervention of child protection agencies, but very unlikely that a parent not sending a child to religious school would be deemed to be an appropriate trigger for a child protection enquiry.

The point is that no matter how 'culturally competent'[4] practice is, the child protection practitioner is the *subject* and the client is the *other*. The otherness of the client is evident even when the professional is himself or herself from a minority community – it is inherent in the professional role. In order to think like a professional at all, individuals must work within the system of thought, and of morality, which is characteristic of Western liberal professionalism. This can cause enormous personal conflict for the individual professional (Gilroy, 1987) but is nonetheless an inevitable part of being a professional in a Western context.

Culturally sensitive practice may well involve an attitude of respect, interest and concern, but there is a level at which professional thought cannot allow the practitioner to pass. A practitioner may be able to describe the world-view of the client, but *qua professional* s/he cannot share that world. This means that practitioners, especially from minority communities, must live with two, possibly incompatible, world-views which they must try to reconcile as best they can. The problem is that the very language in which the arguments are made assumes a certain cultural stance and it is difficult, if not impossible, to transcend this stance. This means that true 'cultural competency', in the sense that Abney and Gunn in their 'Rationale for Cultural Competency' (1993) use the term, is not possible. It may be possible to imagine what it must be like to view the world from a different cultural perspective, but it is not possible to share that 'world-view'.

Finally, the child protection system is, by its very nature, totalizing – i.e. it has the mission to protect *all* children. This means that although it can live with difference in relation to parenting styles, it cannot live with differences in outcomes. Child protection therefore sees different cultural practices as superficial differences of emphasis in parents' attempts to achieve autonomy, independence, equality and happiness for children. Practices that do not have this aim are *ipso facto* morally unacceptable and abusive.

Other cultures in Western humanist thought

One of the characteristics of the humanist literature on culture is that practices in other cultures, usually far away or long ago, are cited in order to refute or confirm the practices that the author intends to promote or attack. Contrast the following examples:

> It is true that, in the past, sexual activity between children and adults was very acceptable in some cultures; however the offender is not living in those cultures, nor will he ever live in those cultures. It may be that…our culture will change, and (such) sexual activities will be acceptable. However, the adult before the courts is not living in a culture of the future, but in the present, and it is the current law that he must be responsive to.
>
> (Abel *et al.*, 1984, p. 100)[5]

> In many Native American cultures, (as well as some African cultures), gay men held honoured status in a tribe, often recognised for having special talents and skills necessary for the survival of tribal members.
>
> (Arey, 1995, p. 201)

These quotations illustrate how the 'other' is subsumed under the moral discourse within Western humanism, not as a subject, but as a mirror for the beliefs of the protagonists. It is clear that these authors are not really concerned with the world-views of the people within the cultures which they cite; these cultures are deployed to further Western political arguments. More importantly, these extracts beg the question of the basis on which the cultural practices of others can be judged – why is it that the belief that adult–child sexual relationships should be sanctioned is labelled as a 'cognitive distortion' whilst the belief that homosexuality can be normal in other cultures is seen as a legitimate argument for the social construction of homophobic attitudes? Of course it is possible to find a society somewhere, sometime which has legitimated almost any human behaviour.

This is further complicated by the fact that 'culture' and 'custom' are often cited as reasons for maintaining practices which *are* unacceptable. Classic examples of this are foot-binding in Chinese culture and *Suttee* in Hindu culture. The carrying of 'cultural weapons' by Zulus in South Africa, and Orange marches through Catholic areas of Northern Ireland are other examples where culture and tradition are used as excuses for intimidation, harassment and abuse of individuals or groups. Thus there is no easy answer to the question of how moral judgements can be made about 'other' cultural practices.

Because of its tendency to deal with difference in a trivial way and to deny its own contradictions, cultural sensitivity has failed to address the real needs of people from minority ethnic communities. The difficulty arises when 'cultural sensitivity' is left conveniently undefined, so that it becomes de facto what the practitioner decides it should be, leaving the victim of culturally sensitive practice confused and disoriented.

Another problem with culturally sensitive practice is that, from the point of view of the 'victim' there is little difference between behaviours or attitudes that are acknowledged to be racist, and behaviour in which racism is disputed. Anti-racist social work texts like those of Jackson (1996), Dominelli (1988) and Cheetham *et al.* (1981), all talk about 'institutional racism'. This is racism which is perpetrated by organizations rather than individuals. Nevertheless, the case examples inevitably boil down to individuals' misunderstanding, incompetence or prejudice, and racism is always seen as an act perpetrated by individuals who are either misinformed or malicious. Thus, in Western culture, difference has been dealt with in two opposing ways – by attacking it or by trying to counsel those who discriminate into accepting the error of their ways. In this respect the quote by Jackson is particularly interesting. Her statement that for people like herself, who do not have those traditions to consider, circumcision is 'barbaric' reveals the true nature of Western liberal thought, which includes anti-racism. She sees herself as unencumbered by cultural traditions, while those from minority communities perversely cling onto traditions which mark them off as more primitive and less enlightened than Western intellectuals, who represent the pinnacle of ethical development.

The fantasy of all these texts is that 'racists', either malicious or misinformed, can be changed into anti-racists by providing them with training. Training consists of three components:

- Changing attitudes so that practitioners are able to understand the feelings of victims
- Providing information which breaks down the stereotypes which cause racist attitudes and behaviour
- Understanding the social and political processes which lead to inequality.

Because anti-racism is basically humanist it is unable to countenance the fact that different groups may have genuinely conflicting world-views. Anti-racist orthodoxy as exemplified by Jackson sees the tensions between professional thinking and that of traditional cultures as arising out of misunderstandings which can easily be explained or negotiated. It may well be, however, that some of these conflicts are the result of fundamentally incommensurable ways of viewing morality in relation to children, ways which are not amenable to 'rational' debate.

Anti-racism and other humanist theories stagger uneasily between the view that all cultures have broadly similar criteria for bringing up children, so that abuse in other cultures can be relatively easily identi-fied and dealt with, and the countervailing view that 'black' people live in a completely different moral world which white people are unable to access.

From a Jewish point of view, anti-Semitism has always taken different forms, and direct attacks have always been complemented by practices which purport to show concern for Jews – as long as they change their cultural practices – 'It's not that you're Jewish that we object to, but that you....' The ellipsis has been filled in at different times by different people since the time of the ancient Greeks (Cantor, 1996). The practice of male circumcision, in particular, has been the site of attacks against Jews since biblical times and has been linked with sexual licentiousness (and abstinence!), moral laxity and even financial impropriety (Dresser, 1997).[6] For Jews, attacks on their cultural practices are often seen not as attacks on the practice per se, but as concealing anti-Semitism.

This perception of hidden racist motivations behind ostensibly rational or even philanthropic intentions is shared by other minority communities. It raises the emotional content of debates, and confuses the issues for both sides. In the majority culture, individual acts are seen as the responsibility of the actor, who is expected to take the consequences for his or her actions. In minority communities, actions by individual actors are often perceived to be shared in some respects by the community as a whole.

As a consequence of this historic legacy, it is tempting for Jews to view the current concerns about circumcision as being tinged with just a hint of anti-Semitism, the more so because circumcision is not merely a cultural affectation, but is seen as representing the core of Jewish identity. The response therefore becomes defensively to explain that the practice is not as harmful as it may seem, and that it does not fall into the definition of 'child abuse'. However, this defensive stance leads to an intellectual dead end.

Arguing in favour of circumcision

One of the problems for those who wish to argue for cultural practices which are considered to be morally dubious is that the ground on which the argument has to take place is itself determined by the liberal humanist agenda. It is difficult to argue from the logical perspective of the 'other'. As a consequence, these arguments usually sound convoluted, defensive and self-justifying. Good examples of this are the arguments put forward to justify arranged marriages in various Asian cultures, or about the empowerment of women in different religious communities.[7] In the case of circumcision, arguments put forward include that it does not really cause distress to the child, that it is medically beneficial and that, although it was dangerous in the past, it is now safe. It is now clear, however, that circumcision is not painless, has no demonstrable medical benefits and can be dangerous or even life-threatening for a small number of children (Money, 1985). These rational arguments based on medical criteria are therefore really smokescreens, and are easily demolished. They are smokescreens because they are essentially defensive, and are intended to persuade liberal gentiles and secular Jews that circumcision is really OK, and that they don't have to worry too much about it. Ultimately these arguments are unconvincing because Jews, Muslims and Africans do not circumcise their children for medical reasons.

The humanist argument, however is also based on assumptions which are never challenged, and which provide an unspoken framework for child protection (and anti-racist) interventions. These include the assumptions that:

- 'health' is the only rationale for impinging on human bodies
- risks to individuals are more important than risks to communities or cultures
- the welfare of individuals is more important than, and in tension with, the welfare of cultures

- consent is the basis for intervention
- human behaviour is ultimately rational, i.e. there is a rational explanation for it, and therefore it is subject to rational interventions; and consequently
- institutions, rites, etc. can be explained by the behaviour, and ultimately the beliefs, of people who participate or practise them
- although the techniques of child-rearing may be different in different cultures, the ultimate aims are the same
- avoidance of physical pain and risk are the cornerstones of child welfare and, conversely, allowing a child to suffer pain or placing a child at risk are inherently abusive acts.[8]

It is this individualized view of harm and abuse, and the focus on events rather than on consequences which lead humanist and anti-racist commentators to conflate practices such as circumcision (which is a cultural rite legitimated as an integral part of a belief system) with, for example, sexual abuse by priests (which is a deviant activity perpetrated by individuals who use their powerful positions to exploit others).[9] In Jackson's book, for example, there is no distinction made between those individuals who feel aggrieved at the institutions of the culture in which they were born, and those who suffer sexual abuse from individuals. This gives the book a decidedly Eurocentric feel to readers from minority communities.

This is not to say that the occasional *Mohel* (ritual circumciser) may not get a sadistic frisson from the act of circumcision, but the institution is not designed to satisfy the sexual lusts of *Mohelim*. Nevertheless, professionals persist in lumping together under the definition of 'abusive' activities which take place in minority cultures and which do not conform to their own moral standards. This argument is not simple however. It is complicated by the fact that feminist literature on child abuse has asserted that although certain practices such as incest may be officially prohibited, they are subtly sanctioned by society in order to maintain patriarchal power. Similar arguments are deployed by anti-racists in relation to institutional racism, which persists despite the proscription of racist acts by individuals. It is the resonance of this argument which makes it difficult for anti-racists such as Jackson to separate individual acts of abuse from cultural practices. The fact that circumcision is seen as perpetuating patriarchal power increases this blurring.

The point is that any defence of circumcision within a humanist paradigm has already conceded the main points, and is therefore bound to fail. The best that can be hoped for is an uneasy truce. Hoffman's book, which is the only in-depth study of circumcision from a secular (liberal) Jewish point of view, notes the agonizing of secular Jews who feel compelled to circumcise their children but see this as harmful. He comes up with a kind of messy compromise – that circumcision should be practised with anaesthetics, under proper medical supervision. The book ends with the implied hope that circumcision will simply evolve away into an egalitarian initiation rite shared by males and females in which no physical impingement on the child's body will take place.

Female genital mutilation and male circumcision

The effects of female genital mutilation (FGM) on women is much greater than male circumcision on men. Over and above the immediate pain and the risks of the operation itself, FGM affects the sexual and reproductive life of the woman, and there is a high incidence of infection and other problems. In fact FGM consists of a range of different operations involving different levels of harm.[10] Unlike male circumcision, FGM is the subject of much international debate and regulation. In the UK it has been prohibited by the Prohibition of Female Circumcision Act 1985. In addition, the words 'genital mutilation', unlike 'circumcision' are certainly 'boo-words'[11] and evoke an instinctive emotional repugnance – you can't be *for* genital mutilation.

In many respects however, the arguments for and against FGM are similar to those in relation to male circumcision. FGM has as long a history, is practised in many cultures (mainly in Africa) and is no less culturally embedded than male circumcision (Dorkenoo and Elworthy, 1992; Lightfoot-Klein, 1989). Although Jews may argue that male circumcision has minimal consequences either psychologically or medically, this is not true for babies, and it is certainly not true for older children and adolescents. The quotation from Mandela above belies any argument that this is a painless rite. In fact, pain and blood are an integral part of the ceremony. Thus it is unlikely that the quantitative differences in the degree of suffering of the child explains the huge differences in interest between FGM and male circumcision in legal, moral and professional discourses. The law, for example, proscribes *all* FGM, no matter how extensive, and does not proscribe *any* male circumcision. The argument that the degree of hurt caused by FGM justifies legal prohibition, whereas in male circumcision the cultural benefits outweigh the hurt to individual children, must therefore be questioned. Freeman (1995) deploys the notion of 'cultural pluralism' (as opposed to monism and relativism) to differentiate morally between male circumcision and FGM. Cultural pluralism addresses moral questions cross-culturally by critically examining the arguments put forward within different cultures for the maintenance of particular practices, and contrasting these with universal conceptions of human need. On this basis he concludes that FGM is immoral but male circumcision is morally defensible.

Another probable explanation for the different legal and professional responses to the two practices is that FGM has become part of the global struggle for women's rights, whereas male circumcision, although still an issue for women, has less immediate consequences because the impact on women is symbolic rather than literal. Also, the perpetrators of FGM are much more 'other' than those of male circumcision. There is also the question of power. Despite the recognition by UK professionals that FGM involves the most vulnerable sector of the population – mainly rural African refugees (Royal College of Nursing, 1994), and the acknowledgement that interventions should take this into account, it is easier to tackle this group than the entrenched hierarchies of Jews and Muslims.

One of the major arguments used by opponents of FGM, along with other disempowering cultural practices in relation to women, is that although these practices are currently part of those cultures, they are not integral to the culture or religion itself, and result from a misrepresentation of the Muslim religion (e.g. Dorkenoo and Elworthy, 1992, p. 13). This line of argument is not available to Jews in relation to circumcision, which is absolutely central to the religion. It also makes opposition to male circumcision much closer to opposing Judaism itself.

Conclusion

I have tried in this chapter to show that the question 'Is male circumcision morally defensible?' is not only difficult and complex, but that it may be impossible in principle to answer. It would be easy, but intellectually lazy, to take a relativist 'culturally sensitive' point of view, and simply assert that circumcision is acceptable for people in whose cultures it is a common practice, but not acceptable within Western liberal societies. This kind of relativism assumes that people live in different, incommensurable moral universes, and that individuals in one culture cannot pass judgement on practices within another culture. This is patently not the case – if it were, then there would be no ambivalence about cultural practices and people would simply fall on one or other side of an easily identifiable dividing line. Cultures (and races) would then become neatly packaged bundles of thoughts, beliefs and practices, blithely maintaining a state of internal consistency whilst remaining impermeable to those outside. In relation to circumcision this argument becomes even more implausible. What is the social group that is supposed to share a common sensibility which is unavailable to Western liberals? It is hard to see why secular Jews (let alone their biblical forefathers who initiated the rite in the first place) should be seen to share a moral universe with Muslims and Africans but not with other Western secular people. It is precisely because *individuals* can live in competing moral universes that there is a problem.

On the other hand it would be just as easy to take a monist position by asserting that all physical harm to children is unacceptable, unless it is done for medical reasons.[12] This argument is more plausible, because it at least has the advantage of being consistent, but the thresholds and criteria would then unequivocally be set by modernist humanism, with little room for cultural diversity. The law would have to ban ear-piercing, scarification, etc. as well as circumcision. In this case Jews would be faced with the choice of giving up Judaism or leaving the jurisdiction – a choice they have had to confront many times in their history (Cantor, 1996).

The choices Jewish parents have to make are also problematic. The argument that cultural continuity can somehow be weighed up against individual pain is not a viable way forward, because there is no benchmark with which to make this measurement. In practice, this is the choice secular Jews have to make, but this is not often perceived, at least on the surface, as a moral choice. It is seen as a choice between the risks of physical damage to the child as opposed to the risks of the child being ostracized from the community and the damage to the community itself.

At present, the position is that a refusal to circumcise a son will effectively exclude him from the community. It may be that sometime in the future Judaism will dispense with circumcision as it has dispensed with, for example, stoning adulterers. This is not an immediate possibility because circumcision is at the very centre of Jewish cultural identity. Abandoning circumcision would also be an admission that the humanist/individualist agenda has successfully colonized the innermost recesses of group identity.

In reality, the present situation will continue – secular Jews will have to make painful decisions, and will have to live with moral ambiguity and the opprobrium of the majority community. But perhaps a wider debate about circumcision will provide a more realistic appraisal of the nature of cultural sensitivity and its relation to protecting

children. In particular, it will expose the modernist/humanist nature of
the child protection/child welfare discourse, and will more clearly
demonstrate the boundaries and limitations of the current assumptions
behind culturally sensitive practice. It may also highlight some of the
ambiguities in the relationships between child abuse and morality.
Could it be possible that some behaviours can be abusive but also
morally defensible?

Notes

1 The current debate in the UK about 'refocusing' children's welfare away
from child protection into family support does not affect this argument.
The debate is about means, not about ends or values, and in this respect
'family support' can be equated to child protection.
2 I am defining a secular Jew as any person who identifies him or herself as
Jewish and who does not believe in divine revelation. This would include
Reform Jews and members of Orthodox synagogues who do not themselves believe in divine revelation. This definition would therefore cover a
wide range of religious practices, but would exclude strictly observant
Jews on the one hand and purely nominal Jews on the other.
3 Interestingly, cultural relativism is not seen in a positive light, and has
controversially been blamed for many child protection mistakes (Dingwall
et al., 1995).
4 Cultural competence is defined by Abney and Gunn (1993, p. 20) as 'the
ability to share the worldview of your clients (or peers) and adapt your
practice accordingly'.
5 This is a quotation from an article aimed at providing practitioners with
the arguments for refuting the distorted cognitions of perpetrators of
child sexual abuse. One of the arguments used by such perpetrators to
justify their paedophilia is that such practices are sanctioned by other
cultures such as the ancient Greeks.
6 The popularity of male circumcision in the USA and the UK has been
traced back to the 1880s when doctors noted the lower prevalence of
venereal disease in Jews. This was wrongly attributed to circumcision,
which was seen as a way of preventing masturbation, which in turn was
seen as the root of virtually all male psychological problems. Thus the
moral debate about circumcision has, until recently, revolved around its
supposed effects on sexual conduct during adolescence rather than the
risks to children.
7 See King (1995), especially the chapter by Afshar for examples.
8 See Freeman (1995) for an in-depth discussion of these issues.
9 See Parkinson (1997).
10 See Lightfoot-Klein (1989) for a fuller description of the practice.
11 See Cranston (1953), cited by Archard, ch. 5, n. 1.
12 See Thorpe and Jackson (1997) for a similar argument in favour of anti-
smacking legislation – i.e. that legislation provides an easily identifiable
common criterion for deciding the threshold of abusive behaviour.

7   Meditations on parental love

The transcendence of the rights/welfare divide

Marinos Diamantides

The decline of 'paternalism' in the welfare state

One of the most disappointing developments in modern Western history is the disenchantment with paternalism – the treatment of vulnerable others *as* vulnerable – that is reflected within the welfare state. The basic feature shared by all kinds of paternalistic ideology or practice – which the welfare state adopts – is the recognition that persons often lack the ability to discern and cater for their own needs. Thus, paternalism justifies opting out from the requirement that civilized actions be governed by the principles of reciprocity, consent and self-determination amongst autonomous beings.

The disenchantment with paternalism broadly encompasses two views. For some, unilateral or 'one-way' actions on behalf of a vulnerable other are justifiable, but only retrospectively, according to its success. Individual parents, lovers, friends and carers may indeed achieve such success with regard to their beloved's immediate needs through a total mobilization of private resources, without a single thought for the future and at the expense of less-beloved others with similar needs. The obvious problem of the modern democratic, capitalist state which also aspired to be a 'welfare state' is that its agents and institutions *cannot* replicate this limited success en masse. It is not feasible to mobilize all public resources for the sake of present, individual needs. Moreover, if the state were to aspire to do so, it would usurp the possibility that such human needs as cannot be addressed from the perspective of social reciprocity may continue to be addressed in contexts where arbitrary, subjective 'one-way' actions of paternalistic generosity are traditionally tolerated: i.e. in parenting, love and, to an extent, medical care.

For others, the problem of paternalist action is of an epistemic and a moral nature, and affects the private and public spheres equally. The philosophy of science now acknowledges that the observer affects what is observed, so that one cannot describe human needs in terms of 'pure objective reality' or claim simply to be responding to such needs. This is because human needs, both individually and in their inter-relationship, are not accessible in terms of pure 'objective reality'. Rather, the meaning of 'need' is supplied by the individual who detects it, and is qualified by his/her subjective preferences and values. In this sense, paternalistic 'one-way' action becomes the paradigm of intrusive action upon others. When a parent, lover or carer assumes control over a vulnerable other's welfare, the force of their intrusion *cannot* be justified in terms of a principle of 'objective' necessity. Far from being selfless, such actions are motivated by the paternalist person's self-interest to construe the other person 'in their own image' and impute them with the same, value-ridden and subjective views of what is 'needed'. It is therefore preferable that the state should subject the impulse 'to be kind' to the principles of individual autonomy, consent and self-determination. The 'right' of each individual to have their person and body protected from intrusion should override the desires of their parents, lovers or carers. Conversely, permissible paternalistic actions are permissible only if they are conducive to the furthering of the other person's autonomy, as opposed to his/her mere welfare as understood by the actor.

I have emphasized the word 'cannot' in both the views described above to demonstrate what is common to them. In both these positions, despite their differences in perspective, the problem of paternalistic action is discussed in terms of an implicit promise, and a corresponding power or ability to 'deliver'. The focus on the ability to deliver assumes that the paternalistic 'one-way' action is a temporary *deviation* from reciprocity and so, that if paternalistic action is to be tolerated at all, it must aim to return to such reciprocity by securing either the beneficiary's retrospective real gratitude or ideal consent. A healthy teenager is thus grateful to his/her parents for having forced him/her as a child to eat vegetables. Further, an injured, unconscious adult who has been operated on in an emergency unit can be anticipated to consent to this in retrospect. That is, s/he may not necessarily be expected to agree that the steps taken by the physician were absolutely essential to save his/her life (the patient may not value his/her life), but s/he can at least be expected to agree that the physician undertook measures that s/he honestly believed were prerequisite for the patient's future exercise of autonomy.

Paternalism as 'gift': an expression of higher *parental* desire

However, there is a different perspective. For instance, the philosopher Emmanuel Levinas (1986, pp. 345–59) describes actions of parental care and love in terms of 'gift-giving', a process in which the giver does not anticipate, in fact shuns, any gratitude and/or retrospective authorization by the receiver. The act of gift-giving is ineluctably a *one-way act*; in other words the gift is presented by the giver without any expectation of return in the form of thanks, recognition or gratitude. Such actions indicate the possibility of a 'radical generosity' on the part of the giver. They also indicate the possibility of a particularly 'heteronomous experience' of the receiver by the giver as totally 'other'. So the giver takes it upon him/herself to act for the benefit of the other prior to identifying the needs of the other; and the impetus to act also occurs prior to understanding the other as a distinct, autonomous subject of rights.

Here I wish to approach the issue of paternalistic action from such a perspective. First, the value of paternalistic action will be understood not by measuring its ability to 'deliver' to the actual person at the receiving end, but instead as a form of 'impulsive investment' which is made blindly with regard to the present and past *for the sake of a possible future*. Second, if we are to understand paternalistic actions and decisions as distinct from self-interested ones, we must be able to assert that this 'impulsive' investment is also 'profitless' for the paternalist, in so far as his/her experience of being paternal actually modifies his/her sense of self and cancels any expectation of gratitude. The term 'parentalism' must, at this point, be substituted for 'paternalism'. This is necessary because, traditionally, paternalism refers to the power wielded by (male) progenitors to act upon their offspring in order to ensure that their own past and present will be 'continued' or replicated in their children's future.

In order to distinguish between parentalism and paternalism, let us think about medical care, a situation in which the need for parental action often arises, and in which parental action is frequently indistinguishable from so-called 'medical paternalism'. By the latter we mean the attitude of doctors who treat the patients as 'children' and impose on them a therapy according to what they feel is in the patients' best interests. However, there may still be a genuine parental attitude concealed under this paternalism, for the carer views the patient as *more* than a cluster of present needs that can or cannot be objectively/subjectively known and addressed. The invalid is more than the subject of a subjective experience of pain and discomfort; and s/he is also more than the object of medical scientific knowledge.

What inspires the doctor is love and compassion for the excessive *vulnerability* of each sick person. This vulnerability consists of undergoing suffering whose significance is *future*. For the sufferer this means that s/he suffers more than s/he ever did (each pain is the worst ever), and beyond any promise of cure or compensation. For the carer it means that s/he must give more than possible at present or more than has ever been possible in the past. Therefore 'suffering' and the care it demands 'open up' the doctor–patient relationship to a *future*. They stand for what overwhelms both the sensory capacity of the sufferer (which subjective experience presupposes) and the conceptual or intuitive ability of the carer to empathize with the sufferer's condition. In consequence, the *potential* for caring for the ill logically exceeds the (limited) subjective/objective ability to identify the other's 'needs', and then correlate them with 'what is needed'. The carer feels compelled to offer the other a future which is not yet possible. His/her relationship with the cared-for does not rest on present and past considerations but on a future that has to be imagined and fought for. More generally, the concern for the vulnerable other rests on a desire to face the ill as otherwise-than-ill, i.e. as unique sufferers – not cases of generic pathology – and separate from the illness which pacifies them.

Fecundity

This work of loving and parental care is related to Emmanuel Levinas's pedagogic 'idea of child', expounded mainly in his book *Totality and Infinity* (Levinas, 1969). As the aimless caressing of the beloved indicates, love is not only aiming at an object which can be unavailable or be lost; in caressing one's beloved partner, one encounters the incomparable other, who lies outside of the lovers' past and present, in a future 'not yet'. Hence love incorporates the idea of 'fecundity' through which relationships of love and care relate to the future by being 'impregnated' with the possibility of giving birth to child. Parental love thus begins prior to the existence of a child. Further, it leads to a relationship in which parents do not only 'possess' children but in which, simultaneously, they 'are' their children. In their relation to the idea of 'child' each parent's ego is not destroyed, although it does become 'a stranger to itself'. Parental love is thus elevated to a higher principle – that of governing total transcendence of the self but without loss of identity.

The subject/object divide is radically subverted in the idea that one can actually relate to the other person both as different and as part of one's self by imitating parenthood. To stick with my initial terminology, the decision to become (and the action of becoming) a parent is the archetypal 'one-way action' or donation of a gift for which no gratitude is expected. It is a form of 'blind' but also 'profitless' investment. It is an act of selfless love which nevertheless does not impoverish the giver (it merely gives him/her no extra dividends) and does not belittle the taker (since the taker is not there at the start).

In conceiving the idea of 'child', the 'adult' (irrespective of his/her will and/or ability to conceive biologically), is not merely attempting to duplicate him/herself, but is opening up to the idea of infinity. The future which the child represents and which the parents conceive escapes the logic of continuity from past and present. 'Fecundity' is the relation of the self called 'adult' with itself as stranger. In the actual feeling of parental love (which is to be found in every human who cares for another) the adult comes to transcend the realm of the possible and to respond to a future 'not yet' which, nevertheless, matters to him/herself now.

The progressive duty of parental desire

How does parental love work? Is this one-way act of giving love, which is a response to no specific need on the part of the loved, a duty? 'Need' is an economical notion and so the cogent response it occasions also obeys the economical prioritizing of human needs in any given social order. In today's society one is likely to accept, for example, that stopping a wound bleeding has priority over giving verbal comfort; that infertility and its psychological impact are more significant for a married woman than an unmarried one; that the loss of vision is prioritized over the loss of the other senses.

However, the idea of the other human being as being part of myself, and yet irreducible to my knowledge and experience, allows me to transcend the given order of prioritized needs. The child-loving subject becomes a 'stranger to himself' in the sense set out above, and so becomes free from what is accepted as a given order of identified and hierarchically organized human needs. In this case the substantive choices one makes are informed, either consciously or unconsciously, by *different* forms of knowledge of suffering and experiences of caring than, say, the scientific one, which today constitutes the major paradigm. These may be actual knowledge and practices which emerge from different cultural settings; or they may be past ones from the same cultural setting which have been superseded and marginalized by modern approaches. (For instance, the religious approach to illness has been superseded by the scientific one, but continues to be of importance to some individuals and communities.)

Thus, the desire to approach the other person as 'child' allows the subject of parental love to respond to his/her needs from a point of view in which accepted priorities can be challenged and in which forgotten ones can be given new priority. Working with marginalized or obsolete human 'needs' is not nostalgic, but puts these needs to use for an even more radically different *future*. As a result, one can make 'surprising' subjective choices as to what is 'needed'. Traditional Western parents may decide to reject medical advice for an operation on their child – where the child has already been operated on 'more than enough' – in a way that makes them resemble Eastern Buddhist parents. In reverse, a Buddhist person living in Britain may decide that, although s/he would usually disdain the Western obsession with beauty, at least when it comes to their beloved, 'hair loss' is important and treatment should be sought. What allows them to care in this way by 'transcending' themselves and the present, and putting the past to the service of the future? In their desire to satisfy their parental love, the subjects of that love effect a kind of *reshuffling* of the order of natural needs which they would otherwise find neatly organized in their specific cultural domain. This compassion, which frees the carer to reorder priorities, is what has been described here as the vocation of parental love.

Good and bad parenting

It is often assumed that respect for a minor person's rights, which views the minor as a unique individual capable of exercising autonomy and not as 'one more child with a child's needs', is antithetical to the tendency of adults to treat children 'paternally', i.e. as dependent yet separate others. I would argue, however, that the imputation of rights to minors is motivated by the same parental desire which propels concern for their welfare. Only if we realize how inescapable 'parental desire' is, will we be able to accept that our decisions and actions with regard to minors (and, for that matter, any other human being whose welfare is in danger) can never be 'cleansed' of their ineluctable, 'one-way' force. Any attempt to pre-empt our irreducible responsibility by prior understanding as to whether the minor is presented to us either as a dependent entity or as an autonomous being, will mask the fact that it is the adult's love which conceives the child as both an internal and an external entity.

Actual parents address their child as *both* an autonomous human being *and* as a child like others. Modern liberal parents often assume their children are unique from a very early stage; often new parents act as if they are actually having a conversation with an infant who can barely utter a word. This imputation of uniqueness is necessary for the enjoyment of their child as a separate human being. When children are seen as distinct beings they offer exceedingly good company. But this imputation is seldom the dry product of logic: parents speak to their child, ask him/her what it wants, and so on, with incredible passion. They know that at this stage the child is not yet more than a 'cluster of needs', yet they continue to treat what has barely left the womb as if it were unique, 'the only child of its kind'. By imputing a minor with autonomy, adults envisage him/her as a human being who is *external* to them and not an entity 'in their possession'. However, parents also see their offspring as 'their only' child, the child they cannot allow to die. As a result, depending on the dangers that the child faces if left to its own devices, the parents will also be ready to contradict their child's autonomy and treat their son or daughter as part of themselves, as a possession whose needs must be addressed resolutely, because a threat to its survival is a threat to them.

Parents cannot afford to make an artificial division between minors as autonomous 'subjects of rights' and minors as objects of welfare concern. They must show patience. If they refuse to accept the minor as a separate other, they can merely *have* children. Parents who care exclusively for the child's welfare but refuse to impute it with autonomy, end up with burdensome children consisting of no more than their many and special needs. Conversely, if parents do not assert their concern for the circumstances of the immature and needy child they have, they will end up *being* their children without *having* any children. The substantive difference between successful and unsuccessful parenting is defined in the simple observation that good parenting creates anew and painstakingly maintains the tentative split between 'child' as autonomous *and* 'child' as dependent; bad parenting simply creates the view of the child as either one or the other. The offspring of good parents will become both autonomous and dependent because his/her parents instructed it to be so. By contrast, the offspring of bad parents will either become an accessory to his/her parents or a 'spoilt child'.

Responsibility and apology

In everyday life, in classrooms and homes, good teachers and good parents simultaneously care for the children 'according to their needs' *and* treat each child as if it is the 'only one of its kind'. They do this by means of a singular 'one-way' act that assumes control over the child and at the same time apologizes for taking this control. The difference between good and bad parenting can also be put in terms of irresponsibility/responsibility for the *kind* of priority of the child's needs that a parent or teacher has adopted, as well as in terms of the presence/absence of apology for the fact that such a choice is not absolute. Good parents do not conceal the mastery and transitivity which characterize their actions towards their children. They may, for instance, decide that eating vegetables is necessary and instruct their child accordingly. At the same time they *apologize* for doing so. They say, 'This is the best I can do for you' or 'This is as much as I know.' Bad parents, by contrast, claim false authorities for whatever they resolve to do. The child who is forced to eat vegetables not in order to please his/her parents but 'because they are good for you', is swallowing more than courgettes – s/he is swallowing a false 'objective' truth. For s/he hears that 'eating vegetables is good for you', which in fact means that eating vegetables is good for 'children' as a category: the child's autonomy has already been dealt a mortal blow. Telling the child that 'it does not matter' if it does not eat any vegetables is another false truth. Successful parenting requires saying 'please, please me by eating your vegetables so I can feel that you are OK'.

The distinction I draw between successful and unsuccessful parenting on the basis of the degree of responsibility is not merely of theoretical interest. Psychologists and psychoanalysts make a living out of treating symptoms caused by the absence of the former or the presence of the latter in children's early development. Nor is it simply of interest to (actual or potential) biological parents. Often the parental attitude is at play in relationships between children and adults who must make decisions on children's affairs. Here, I will concentrate on responsibility for the desires of children in child law by analysing specific judgements in which the judges adopt parental concern but fail to apologize for it.

The Gillick case

In the 1986 Gillick[1] case in England, the House of Lords passed the landmark decision that a fifteen-year-old girl was entitled to seek advice on and prescription of contraceptives from her doctor even in the absence of parental consent. The case was initiated by the girl's mother, who challenged a government circular which appeared to sanction giving advice on contraception in the absence of parental consent. The Lords' decision overruled the opposite conclusion reached earlier by the Court of Appeal and upset a centuries-old common-law view of minors, simply on the basis of their status as 'minors', as incompetent to consent to (or, alternatively, refuse) medical treatment.

This decision has been greeted warmly by commentators as something of a landmark for children's autonomous rights. But of course there is the view that a 'child' should not only be thought of as an 'adult-like' entity, but also as a vulnerable other who often finds him/herself over-exposed to whatever there is 'out there': a child is not master of his/her world. The very idea of a child in danger is so repulsive that danger must be separated from the child. The child's bystander must become its parent – at once separate from it and united with it, a complete stranger and also a part of him/herself. The old law, which the medical profession had interpreted to mean that children could give no valid consent to medical treatment before their sixteenth birthday, but that they could give consent immediately after that day, was not only 'unrealistic', but contrary to the principle of self-determination. The decision should not be seen as part of a trend to render children 'adult-like'. The decision did not mean that from then on all minors were automatically to be construed as autonomous and capable of defying their parents in deciding issues of medical treatment.

The significance of such a decision is more than a second-stage clarification of an abstract point of law in a high court. This legal decision, like any other, should not merely 'develop' or 'amplify' legal doctrine, rather it must create or 'give birth' to *totally new law* inspired by new and different circumstances. The former is, of course, possible but in that case judgement is 'still-born' (Diamantides, 1995). Assuming this framework, the judges in the Gillick case had to be capable of conceiving genuinely new law on children out of simple parental impulse. However, in the event, the birth of the 'Gillick child' (i.e. the new way of conceptualizing in law the idea of 'child' suggested by the case), to view it metaphorically, was a healthy labour leading to an unwanted child for whom the parents will not take responsibility.

Responsibility would have been taken if the judges in the Gillick case had explicitly endorsed the tensions between the idea of children's rights and the concern for their welfare. In reality the law continues to be that a minor can, independently of the opinion of its parents, seek medical advice on contraceptives, if – and this is an important if – the minor is evidently capable of using them properly, where 'properly' includes 'when it is good to use them' (according to adults). In short, the judgement contains no grand resolution of the welfare–rights divide, but instead maintains the tension. However, it does not passively replicate the problem because the judgement also performs a pedagogical role. It teaches a certain lesson as to the *manner* in which parental discretion over minors' welfare ought to be exercised. By saying that the autonomy of minors must be presumed by adults and only then rebuffed (if at all), the judgement – and this is the true moment of judicial creativity – subjects adult discretion over minors' welfare to an ever-greater degree of responsibility for the welfare priorities and choices they impose on minors, even (or especially) when exercised in the best of faith.

The importance of this responsibility can be stated in terms of my earlier phraseology in which parental action was taken to be radically 'one-way'. Levinas also describes this radically open action as a 'departure without return' (1986, p. 349) or as a gift given to the other as *other* to my experience and knowledge, therefore other than the needs with which I identify him/her (and so objectify him/her), and other to my knowledge of him/her as a separate being, which rests on a logical presupposition of difference and individuality (through which I subjectify him/her). This other cannot merely be the external object of my concern or the abstract presupposition of a subject in my mind. However, this 'departure without return' that is parental love can

> lose its absolute goodness if the work sought for its recompense in the immediacy of its triumph.…[T]he one-way movement would be inverted into a reciprocity. The work, confronting its departure and its end, would be absorbed again in calculations of deficits and compensations, in accountable operations.…The one-way action is possible only in patience, which, pushed to the limit, means for an agent to renounce being the contemporary of its outcome, to act without entering the promised land.
>
> (Levinas, 1986, p. 349)

In the Gillick appeals the various judgements can each be seen as addressing the 'idea of child' and providing a lesson on good parenting. Each judgement accepts the inevitability of 'one-way' actions; but each judgement also informs us that in every case parental concerns must accommodate respect for children's rights. This double requirement can be met, I would argue, only in a *radically* 'generous' manner in which the 'one-way' action does not hide its unilateral character. That is, one has to assume personal responsibility for one's 'one-way' actions of parental love aiming at the other's vulnerability and not by claiming any false truth or authority. One who does not want to be seen as 'subjective' or 'arbitrary' but who hides in his judgement behind claims of 'doing what is necessary' does not care for the other. When applied to actions and decisions aimed at particular children's needs, what one is obliged to say is that one 'took the liberty' of conceiving of the children in the abstract as *both* objects of concern *and* as subjects of rights in such a way that one could 'reshuffle' the children's needs from one's privileged 'superior' position.

The judges, however, ultimately failed in their pedagogic role towards parents, carers and all adults who at various instances have to assume responsibility for children. The judges – typically for modern judges – assumed the role of impersonal 'agents of the law'. Similarly, they invited everyone else to justify their impositions on children on the basis of an 'objective test' for children's maturity. What the judges in this case did was to shift the focus of the legal test for determining the competency to receive contraceptive advice from the child's status (i.e. minority) to his/her actual 'capacity to understand'.

The test of this capacity became one in which the minor has to show that s/he understands the purpose and effects of the medical treatment sought against the will of his/her parents. This 'test' is supposedly capable of measuring a child's maturity in an objective yet individual manner. However, the notion that maturity as 'a manifestation and reflection of the minor's physiological, psychological and environmental influences' is *objectively measurable* inverts the significance of responsible parental 'one-way' action (Levinas, 1986). In Levinas' words, the one who rests his/her action for a vulnerable other on the grounds of an objective or subjective necessity is effectively seeking a 'recompense in the immediacy of' its triumph of objectivity, and so his or her work appears based on calculations of deficits and compensations. In this case the sought-after triumph was that of impartiality and objectivity in representing a child who is mature. But today's claim of triumph is tomorrow's defeat. In a subsequent case involving an anorexic child the same 'objective' test was effectively put aside, since the judges felt that the mere presence of certain important psychological and/or physiological needs (such as those of an anorexic teenager[2]) cancels the dilemma between children's rights and their welfare, and transforms the child into an object of concern. What this suggests is that the outcome of the court's testing of a minor's 'actual' degree of maturity is not objective but simply represents the judges' preference for certain signs of maturity.

In the Gillick case only one thing is certain. The judges, faced with the idea of 'child', asserted that children's autonomy cannot be brushed aside. Nevertheless children's autonomy (like all autonomy) must be seen as an adult abstraction and imputation to minors. It does not cancel children's dependency or the adults' parental duty to treat them *as* dependent by assuming mastery, control and transitivity. It rather acts as a guarantee that, irrespective of what one does for a child, one has to apologize to the child *as if* it was autonomous. The possibility of facing a dependent child and yet apologizing as if that child was autonomous is no less than the effect of the idea of the child as transcendent on the adult. As I have stated earlier (p. 112) this idea transcends the subject–object divide and allows an adult to become a stranger to him/herself and yet retain his/her own identity. Parental love is not truly a one-way act, unless it simultaneously addresses the minor as object of concern *and* subject demanding apology.

However, concerning the substantive effects of the Lords' decision in the Gillick case it is difficult to ascertain exactly how the judges 'reshuffled' the hierarchy of children's welfare needs. In the event, priority was given to the need of modern children to have direct access to medical advice on contraceptives over any conflicting needs that biological parents invoke. To a certain (limited) extent the judges acknowledged the subjectivism of their decision by admitting having taken into account the widespread present availability of contraceptives and antiquated anxiety over the independence of the young. However, this acknowledgement does not amount to a full apology, for it is rhetorically presented as a mere 'supplement' to the decision. Apart from that supplementary logic, it was as if the relevant autonomy of children just 'had to be recognized', and, as if the maturity of children is 'objectively' ascertainable.

In this regard, the judges were misleading in presenting their personal instructions as if they were the 'dictate' of impersonal, formal law (one could have relied on formal law in order to arrive at the opposite decision) and/or the result of ascertaining the modern child's 'true' needs. This misleading self-explanation also suggests that it is not easy, today, to justify one's parental attitude publicly. The general problem in the analysis of such a case concerns, therefore, the inability of the judges to express clearly how, in the event, their singular parental subjectivity had assumed mastery over the 'either…or' between, on the one hand, the focus on children's rights and, on the other, the focus on their welfare. In other words, although we can posit that they acted as parents and teachers committed to 'blind and profitless' investments, we can only second guess the type of investment they were making.

What forms of knowledge and what different experiences of children's vulnerability did the judges rely on in reaching their decision? We can only speculate.

In any case, what remains of the Gillick judgement, once it is stripped of its pretensions to objectivity and realism, is a sense of *bad* parental talk of the 'magisterial' type in which the force of parental adult action for children is obscured and mystified. Good parental talk requires *personal* responsibility and apology. It requires an exposure of how deep and inescapable the *personal* implication of adults in children's affairs is. What is missing from the Gillick case is the personal communication from parent to child that says 'this is what I can do for you, but it is less than I must'. We are therefore left with a *paternalistic* judgement on children; in other words, one where the judges claimed to speak 'the truth' for the child instead of accounting for their own momentary truth. Here, the role of master and teacher does not deserve the name 'parental love', for the judges failed to acknowledge that 'love' which enabled them to create a new law for children.

Conclusion

Alison Diduck's contribution to this volume (Chapter 8) depicts modern adult anxiety about the indeterminacy of 'childhood' in the form of a double fear. The fear that the recognition of children's rights may result in a parody if children's deep dependency and vulnerability becomes obscured and they are thought to be adult-like; and the fear that without said recognition, adults may forget that today's children are not like yesterday's, that newer possibilities are open to them than were open to us and that different factors challenge their development. I believe these fears to be the causes of good, parental concern. Indeed, if they are not imputed with autonomous rights, children appear inseparable from us, they appear as valuable possessions, as returns on our own life's self-investment. We cannot enjoy the company of children under such circumstances. They weigh on us as much as yesterday's bad purchase. But the recognition of children's rights will by no means crown our desire to enjoy children as at once part of us and other than us with a triumphal end. We shall be always answerable to children for the very work they inspire in us, work which nevertheless cannot be justified by reference to a would-be 'definitive' conceptualization of children. The work of parental love is not responding to objective needs nor can it anticipate retrospective thanks and consent on the part of the future subject it creates. It is essentially a 'one-way' action that no 'bridging' of the rights/welfare divide can do away with.

I started this chapter by referring to the disenchantment with the false promise given by the welfare state that the tension between the desire to address human needs and the determination to impute the vulnerable with autonomy is 'triumphantly' resolvable. Such a triumph would take the form either of the elimination of all the needs which we witness with horror, or of 'compensating' the vulnerable with the ideal assurance that their needs are addressed in an objective order. However, the objective of the counting of human needs is infinite and human suffering is beyond subjective compensation.

We need to put aside the ideality of reciprocity between the weak and their witnesses, and do away with the logic of promises of success or objectivity. We need to remind ourselves that the work of 'goodness' is not anticipating any reward and does not apprehend its object, for it is departure with no return. Parental love is a departure aiming at an abstractly separate, future 'child' which eludes total objectification or subjectification. For the sake of the child's future the parent is *free* to transcend him/herself. New configurations of human needs and vulnerabilities appear, which the parent has not addressed as yet. The demand is never-ending, as is the freedom to take responsibility for 'one-way' actions.

Towards the end of this chapter I turned to the state and specifically to the institution of law. The problem with law's intervention in children's welfare is not that it artificially rids children of their vulnerability by imputing them with an 'adult-like' autonomy. Imputing children with autonomy does not (and could not) undermine the parental freedom of adult subjects to provide for their children's welfare. The imputation of rights merely highlights the high risk of the 'blind and profitless' investment – the 'one-way' movement of love and concern from adult to child – being reversed towards seeking reciprocity and a loss of its absolute goodness. This risk materializes when it is revealed that the investor has in fact 'foreseen' or anticipated the child s/he invested in. This foreseeing attempts to arrest the otherness of childhood either in an adult-like autonomous subjectivity or in an absence of subjectivity. Yet, the treatment of children as distinct beings despite their dependency is no less than a prerequisite for the possibility that each child's welfare needs will be conceived of and ordered in a fresh manner, both at the cost and the freedom of great personal responsibility. The Gillick case goes to show that the individuals who pass for 'agents' of the welfare state – judges included – enjoy the same freedom as parents. But the case also shows that they do not, as yet, pay the same personal price.

Notes

1 *Gillick v West Norfolk and Wisbech Area Health Authority* (1986) AC 112.
2 *Re J (A Minor): Medical Treatment* (Court of Appeal, 10 July 1992).

8   Justice and childhood

Reflections on refashioned boundaries[1]

Alison Diduck

Law and justice

> Law and justice are at best distant cousins...
> (Marlon Brando in *A Dry White Season*)

This popular, sceptical, understanding of law as in some way distant from justice roughly coincides with the way that lawyers themselves see the relationship between the legal and the moral. Lawyers' justice (as the above quotation implies) does not rely exclusively upon judgements as to the 'rightness' or 'wrongness' of behaviour, but resides also in such principles as equal treatment before the law, consistency between similar cases and compliance with correct procedures. Indeed, the application of these legal principles often leaves little space for moral judgements, and when they do occur, they are likely to be seen by judges as falling outside the legal realm.[2] In order to further pursue this dichotomy between law and morality and their differing notions of justice, it is important to examine the *legal subject*, that is the image that law creates and conveys of those people who come to or are governed by law. In the Anglo-American liberal tradition, law tends to convey the image of people as autonomous, rational and self-interested individuals. It is this image which then becomes generalized and universalized as *the legal subject*. Legal subjects are assumed to know their own mind and to act in their own interests. The law is not usually required to consider their welfare. It is the subject's rights and freedoms which are the major concerns of the law.

In other conceptions of justice which have been said to lie somewhere outside law, however, perhaps in the realm of morality or religion, the individual's subjectivity may be understood slightly differently.[3] In this realm, the subject may bear a connection to others or duties to others. Justice for this subject is concerned with his or her welfare and the well-being of the others with whom he or she is connected. Recently, debate around this moral subject has begun to inform law, such that any artificially constructed boundaries between it and the legal subject are being revealed as illusory. The moral duties to others and connections with others that traditionally have not been recognized in the law made for the autonomous individual[4] may thus be included in a *newly* understood process of 'doing justice'.[5]

If, then, we are able to break down boundaries between legal and moral subjectivities, we can go further and suggest that justice for those subjects may cross those boundaries as well. Justice may, for example, require attention both to people's welfare and to their rights, to both their dependence and independence. An integrated 'justice' in this sense may also accord more readily to our 'everyday experience as practical members of real social [legal] worlds' (Jenks, 1996, p. 12) in which we live as women, men and children dependent upon *and* independent of one another. Law's failure to recognize this type of integrated justice means too often that '[l]aw dresses us with a veneer of rights, duties and responsibilities (legally conceived) that have nothing to do with real needs and attributes of human beings' (Norrie, 1993, p. 13).

The problem is that a reconception of the legal subject that takes account of its connections to others and to its situation, and a reconception of legal justice that recognizes the conditions and relationships of connection may seem to be a violation of those very liberal principles of equality and universality upon which modern Western law is based. For able-bodied adult males, whose subjectivity rests comfortably within the liberal autonomous tradition, it may cause particular problems. For others, however, particularly for children, the problems may be fewer. It may be easier to incorporate a reconstituted child subject into an integrated notion of legal justice. Children's subjectivity, while seemingly and traditionally fixed within the moral realm of dependence and connection, is currently facing a 'crisis' which has not directly confronted adult subjectivity. While childhood has always been an elusive concept, only acquiring its modern and universal meaning in relatively recent times (Hendrick, 1990), the current 'crisis' of childhood has forced us to rethink again what childhood means. The implications for yet a further reformulation of the meaning of childhood, however, go beyond understandings of justice for children. If the boundary that divides a universal notion of childhood from that of adulthood can be seen as permeable, it becomes less compelling to cling to the understanding of adult subjectivity as fixed and immutable. Finally, it may become easier to see boundaries between law and morality as equally open to question.

Constituting the subject

There is nothing new in the suggestion that childhood is not a natural category – it is a social, legal, political, economic and moral construction which always relates to a particular cultural or temporal setting.[6] In more ways than this, though, it is a relational construct. First, as an identity or a category it requires an opposition, a contrast. Children are that which adults are not. More than that, they are what adults are not now, but once were, that which adults have grown, developed or matured *from*. Childhood, according to this view, is seen as a separate stage (Archard, 1993, p. 30). In this understanding we see a process of metamorphosis informed by the idea of evolution or progression: the primitive developing through stages into ultimate maturity (Jenks, 1996, p. 9; Archard, 1993). Children are, in this sense, qualitatively different from adults (Hendrick, 1990, p. 42), as established in the 1830s debates about the 'nature' of a child being different in kind from that of an adult (Hendrick, 1990, p. 42), but they are also incomplete adults. Further, sociologist of childhood Chris Jenks argues that the postwar dominance of theories of moral, cognitive and psychosexual development, and of a particular understanding of the phenomenon of socialization means that eventual adulthood comes to be perceived almost as the sole purpose of childhood (Jenks, 1996). In this sense, and in light of 'common sense' which suggests characteristics of immaturity or childishness (such as dependence, vulnerability, cognitive or moral immaturity) are defects in adults, children are also inadequate adults; they have not yet achieved that level of maturity which makes them fully socialized persons (Jenks, 1996).[7]

Child and adult remain radically different from one another, the one being definable only by reference to, or in opposition to, the other. One can see this relationship as an interdependence (Archard, 1993, p. 161). Another way to look at it may be that in their separation or opposition lies not only their difference, but also their intimate connection. 'A mode of relation that is oppositional still assumes a prior presence of identity that goes out from or asserts itself' (Fitzpatrick, 1998, p. 26). While the adult 'self' excludes the child we once were, and adult conceptions of childhood exclude our adult 'selves', both retain fragments of the other identity, fragments similar to that which Fitzpatrick calls 'insistent residue' (Fitzpatrick, 1998). It is the opposition yet 'intimate connection' (*ibid.*) of the boundaries between childhood and adulthood that I would like to explore, suggesting that it is analogous to intimate connections between different notions of justice.

Childhood, however, is also relational in another sense – the sense that because it is the state at which people have not yet completed their progress towards adulthood, their development, they are vulnerable and still connected to another, socially, psychologically, economically and emotionally (Jenks, 1996, p. 40). The child is *dependent*. Indeed, dependence was seen as a crucial identifying characteristic of childhood when the current definitional boundary was being formed. In nineteenth-century debates about juvenile delinquency, independence was seen as contrary to the state of childhood. Dealing with delinquency involved bringing the child 'to a sense of dependence by re-awakening in him new and healthy desires which he cannot himself gratify' (Hendrick, 1990, p. 44). Increasingly dominant discourses of psychology and health promoted developmental theories, according to which adulthood is now seen to be attained after a long process of maturation. It is the state in which one achieves the highest levels of psycho-social, cognitive and moral development; it is individuation, achievement of independent selfhood, autonomy and rationality. It occurs after a process during which the child sheds its dependence to become autonomous and independent. It is a process only at the *end* of which, on achieving selfhood, one is invested with a subjectivity which is readily understood as a *legal* subjectivity, that which encompasses autonomy and rationality. Justice for those who have attained that level of development – adults[8] – is achieved by protecting this autonomy, usually in the form of rights. Justice for those who have not attained an autonomy deemed worthy of protection – children – must come from something different, but something which must also protect the integrity of their subjectivity as we understand it. Justice for children is achieved, therefore, by protecting their dependence, usually in the guise of their welfare. Autonomy/rights and dependence/welfare are therefore deemed almost incompatible, the one set attributed to a constructed adult identity, and the other set to a constructed child identity.

But children's dependence and welfare have particular characteristics. The primary one is their association with a child's carers, and the role those carers adopt in sustaining the child's dependence and ensuring his or her welfare.[9] When justice for children comes to be determined by law, then, law must incorporate these relational notions of dependence and welfare which are rooted in historical and cultural understandings of adult–child relationships, particularly the mother–child relationship. In fact, children embody the irrevocable dependency relationship; when we look at children we see also the parent, most usually the mother (Jenks, 1996, p. 42). Mother is perceived as 'natural' nurturer, or 'natural' caretaker who bears a relationship with her child which seems to be explicable only in terms of 'maternal instinct' or mystical or biological bonds forged in the womb or early infancy. In this view, mother and child are not quite a unit, but neither are they quite separate (Diduck, 1999). They are a unit/not-unit with a subjectivity which contrasts sharply with the legal subjectivity of the autonomous individual. Their relationship is based upon 'love' or 'maternal bonds', and this is antithetical to the liberal legal relationship based primarily upon relations of rights or of exchange (Diduck, 1999). Explanations for this connection between mother and child have taken different forms, from the maternal feminism of both nineteenth- and twentieth-century feminists to the views of anti-feminist commentators which explain women's connection with children in terms of women's capacity for intuition and empathy, and their incapacity for reason and rationality (Cox, 1996).[10]

Others take a social constructionist position focusing upon social, economic and political conditions to explain the connection as literally man-made,[11] and point to the often patriarchal conditions in which the mother–child relationship appears to be natural. Women's political confinement to the private sphere is one of those historical conditions, as is the sexual division of labour which continues to be based upon it.[12] Despite (or because of?) the conditions in which mothering is done, 'mother embodies dependency at the same time that she is trapped by the dependency of others, marred by burdens of obligation and intimacy in an era where liberation and autonomy are revered' (Fineman, 1995, p. xi). She is connected to her child who embodies the 'flip side' of her dependency. Childhood and motherhood, then, epitomize in current understanding relational or connected subjectivities different from the autonomous subjectivities required and assumed by law. They are therefore protected through a moral discourse of caring (Smart, 1991) or welfare rather than a legal discourse of rights and exchange.

In this way, children as subjects emerge from a particular structuring and understanding of social relationships, and the meaning we attribute to childhood derives from the forms of discourse that accompany those relationships, including ideologies of motherhood and care, and notions of need and dependency (Jenks, 1996). Through these discourses, a child becomes the best example of the embodiment of a connected, interdependent subject. Unlike adult subjectivity, this intimate and dependent subjectivity is difficult for liberal notions of justice to accommodate, based as they are on abstracted autonomy, independence and disconnection from other subjects and social conditions. Some explain the result of this incongruity as law treating children as 'legal objects' rather than as legal subjects (Freeman, 1983). Others (*ibid.*; Archard, 1993) suggest that children's subjectivity *ought* to be invested with some degree of adult-like legal subjectivity so that law's justice can accommodate them. Still others, including myself, suggest that the answer may lie as much in the radical reformulation of 'the adult' and of justice as much as of the child. Short of such a radical change, children may possess a kind of legal subjectivity, but it is one which must first be comprehended in a moral/ethical register before it can be expressed in a legal one, and so the language of welfare and care is adopted by the same law which usually speaks of rights and autonomy. The ill-fit of individual children within this language can easily result in unjust outcomes for them. An example of this might be laws which mandated the wholesale removal of aboriginal children from their families in both Canada and Australia, and their placement with 'white' families: activities which were said to be undertaken in the interests of the children (Monture, 1989).

Let me take the notion of the ill-fit further, along the lines of the ill-fit between the 'veneer' law gives us and our 'needs and attributes as human beings'. Children and mothers are moral/ethical subjects; childhood and motherhood are emblems of altruism and care, a 'symbol of all that is decent and caring about a society' (Jenks, 1996). But just as it is the *idea* of the autonomous individual which is protected by formal law (Naffine, 1990), so it is the *idea* of motherhood (Yngvesson, 1997; Diduck, 1998) and the *idea* of childhood which are understood morally so as to be protected materially, politically and legally at the expense of everyday mothers and children.

> Children are the keepers of our dreams. They carry in them all our unlived lives. In a country in which many still go without homes or food, it is clear that it is the 'idea' of children which holds our concerns, if not children themselves.
>
> (Harrison, 1991, p. 267)

When individual mothers or children become a matter for legal concern, justice may become lost in the ill-fit between the *idea* of them and the *reality* of their everyday conditions. Excluded from law in these ways, but fitted within it when individual children 'act like' adults, children can be seen not only as the 'interface between politics and psychology' as Donzelot suggested (Jenks, 1996, p. 97), but also as the interface of ethical, political, social and legal relations.

As I inferred earlier, however, whatever we say about children or childhood is 'not altogether really about children and childhood' exclusively: childhood is 'the causal repository for explanation of self' (Jenks, 1996, p. 69) and social and moral relationships, and self and legal relationships. My project, then, is premised upon the idea that how we constitute and understand childhood may help to explain how we constitute and understand self/adulthood and, further, that any insights gained from that understanding may be useful in bridging or filling the apparent gap between the two and also between legal and moral notions of 'justice'. So, my project is about more than children as legal or moral subjects, it is also about adults and about any connections between the two, and between the constitution of subjects and ideas of justice and welfare.

'Potentialities and perils'[13] of reformulated subjectivities

I make no claims about any inherent or inevitable political dangers or otherwise of this concept of childhood as the interface of the relational/moral and the autonomous/legal, other than to note at this point three possibilities. The first is that reliance upon moral or ethical relations of care and welfare which childhood implies, to the exclusion of the protections provided by hard-won struggles for rights, may create injustice by means of exclusion from social, civil or political society. Moral concern can easily turn to moral condemnation, particularly in a political context in which the rhetoric of morality trips off the tongues of both the new right and new labour communitarian left.[14] The Bulger tragedy in which a toddler was killed by two ten-year-old boys is a good example of how the law becomes an arena for moral condemnation. The convicted children, Thompson and Venables, were labelled as 'monsters' and subjected to a barrage of verbal abuse from bystanders as they were brought to and from court during their trial. Further, in a social context in which dependency takes on a 'sinister' meaning (Jenks, 1996, p. 42),[15] protection of children through the ideology of care can become morally approved control of them (Jenks, 1996).[16]

The second possibility is the converse of the first. Reliance upon unreconstructed 'adult' legal subjectivity without accommodating any notions of dependence or welfare for the (child) subject may also result in injustice. Once again, the Bulger case is illustrative in its treatment of apparently uncomprehending ten-year-old children presented as 'adults' in law, at least for the purpose of the criminal trial. If, however, the subjects adult and child are indeed intimately connected, perhaps it is possible to transcend the dichotomies which create their definitional boundaries and their links with morality/legality and dependence/independence respectively. This leads me to the third possibility.

We may be at a moment, politically, when something is happening at the interface of relations I referred to earlier. The previously understood and comfortable category 'childhood' and the moral subject identity of the child are being disrupted, not least by children themselves in their everyday lives. This disruption, or crisis, is forcing a 'radical renewal' (Ashe, 1995) of the child subject either by the renegotiation of the boundaries which create it or by the revelation that these boundaries were mythical in the first place. I am suggesting here an emerging social and political anxiety about disrupted understandings – the challenging of cherished beliefs – which may result in either a crude type of backlash – a retrenchment to reinforce old boundaries (witness the political rhetoric of the first potentiality coming from a not so romantic nostalgia about childhood innocence) – or in continuing new reconceptualizations of childhood. This alternative, third possibility has enormous implications for children's welfare and rights, but may also assist reconceptualizations of the self, and of social, legal and ethical relationships, as well as, finally, of ways to understand moral-legal imperatives such as autonomy, emancipation, dependency, liberation, need, welfare or justice.

On what evidence do I posit this crisis at the interface? How are the categories apparently being dismantled? What phenomena am I talking about?

The crisis of childhood

I see boundaries of meaning being disrupted in part by the 'moral crisis' engendered by apparently increasing numbers of children acting in unchildlike ways. The Bulger case, in particular, forced us to rediscover the fact that children could be violent. Other recent social events also seem to ascribe to childhood an independence, autonomy and self-awareness or self-interest that is irreconcilable with the nature of childhood as we previously understood it. Three notable social phenomena appear to me to be examples of the breach of boundaries between adulthood and childhood. It is interesting also that each appears to be an example of the breach of another 'boundary' – that

128   *Alison Diduck*

between spheres of public and private. I will speculate about the significance of this later.

The first phenomenon is children's increasing activity and power in the market, particularly as consumers (Cunningham, 1995).[17] Children consume directly as well as indirectly in their ability to influence household consumer patterns. Television commercials and children's programmes are aimed at exploiting this influence (Cox, 1996). The identity 'child' is difficult to reconcile with that of 'economic consumer': 'Part of the process of growing up involves learning how to be a consumer, of having money to spend and learning how to make decisions about how to spend it' (Cox, 1996, p. 54).

Children are also producers in the market, albeit more in the 'south' than the 'north' (Bar-On, 1997; Boyden, 1990). Children's engagement with worldly market matters in this way is something which society has not acknowledged since it restricted their participation in paid employment when the current boundaries were first being fashioned. One child protection activist of the early twentieth century, for example, was unable to reconcile the identity 'child' with that of economic producer: 'the term child labour is a paradox – for when labour begins, the child ceases to be' (Cunningham, 1995, p. 144).[18]

In these examples, the image of children as canny economic players disrupts ideas of them as innocents. The public/private boundary breached is that used in a great deal of feminist analysis which posits a distinction between the family as private and the market as public (Olsen, 1983), and is still reflected in domestic and EC law regulating child employment in the public sphere, but not in the private – where it is done for (Bond, 1996) or within the family.[19]

The second condition disruptive to the childhood/adulthood boundary is the Western liberal movement which attributes rights to children, and the consequent ability of children to make rights claims. This movement towards children's rights is substantively different from nineteenth-century demands for children's rights, which meant only the protection of the right to be a child, to be free from responsibilities, and is still remembered legally in the attributed right of a child to play.[20] Late twentieth-century children have many more rights than the right to play, however. Within this new rights consciousness, children are deemed to possess the autonomy and self-consciousness sufficient to be able to make rights claims. Not only can they demand that their human rights be respected by law[21] or claim the right to be heard in legal arenas where decisions about them are being made,[22] they can even initiate proceedings to change their carers.[23] Implicit in the various attempts to promote children's rights is the idea that human dignity and worth come only with rights. This is a position which pays insufficient attention to the dignity and worth that comes with mutual need, interdependence and connection.

A rights-bearing subject is usually assumed to have the capacity of awareness and of understanding of her or his rights and, for them to be of any value, the capacity to enforce those rights.[24] This very unchild-like awareness and calculation of interest crosses the boundary of a different understanding of public/private: a more classical division which sees the public realm as the realm of political citizenship as opposed to the private realm of civil society. Such a move to ascribe legal personality to children in this way implies a rationality, and a degree of political participation and calculation on their part which sit uncomfortably with contemporary principles of welfarism or best interests grown from the paternalistic disempowerment associated with some early children's rights movements.[25]

The third problematic currently facing childhood is children's increasing engagement with what might be termed the 'public sphere' in yet a different way, and that is their increasing and changing engagement with public space. It was social historian Phillipe Ariès who saw the public as the sphere of sociability – the street, the café – as distinct from the private sphere of domesticity – the intensely intimate and increasingly nuclear family (Weintraub, 1990) of mythology if not real life. This distinction has almost been recast into the dangerous and corrupting 'public' *versus* the safe and innocent 'private' (again, relying upon the mythological safety of the family). Outside of parental (maternal) or delegated parental control/protection in which home and school are really the only two proper and safe environments for children, such engagement with the street, the café or, indeed, the shopping mall is considered illegitimate and, like the other illegitimate engagements with the public mentioned above, is seen as a threat to the previously understood concept of childhood. Again, this challenge is not an exclusively modern one but arose also in the nineteenth century as the idea of the modern child was being established (Hendrick, 1990). Its modern manifestation can be seen in the relationship to public space of contemporary street children in 'the south', and in the way that this relationship seems symbolically to disqualify them from being children.

> Qualities admired in adults, such as independence or wariness [which children learn on the street] are therefore generally frowned upon in children....[The delinquent or street child] can take care of his own immediate interests...[and] asks for no

protection. He has consequently much to unlearn – he has to be turned again into a child.

(Hendrick, 1990, p. 43)[26]

Alison Young (1996) also speaks of the dissonance between the inappropriate public child and the appropriate private one. She highlights the publicized pictures of Robert Thompson and Jon Venables in their school uniforms – their private and appropriate *semblance* contrasted with the *reality* of them outside school, in a shopping centre, unattended (unprotected or uncontrolled) by an adult – engaging with the public space in a way normally reserved for adults (or men at least). This dissonance, as does each of the previous examples, means not only that boundaries between acceptable and unacceptable childhood behaviour are violated, but also that those very boundaries which define childhood itself – that is as *not adulthood* – become perceived as violated or, even more threateningly, as malleable and questionable. In violating so tragically the *idea* of childhood as well as the boundary which creates it, Thompson and Venables almost ceased to be children; they became monsters to some, adults to the law.

In the context of so many apparently unchildlike children, understandings of the concept of childhood become open to interpretation; children's dependence, privateness or connectedness is no longer either taken for granted or (as in the rights example) always assumed to be acceptable (Jenks, 1996). Preserving our sense of what childhood *is* and consequently what justice for children *means* when the boundaries which constitute them are blatantly being broken, therefore, becomes highly problematic. It creates for liberal notions of justice an enigma or, worse, a crisis that has been faced only in different contexts in the past. For example, at the time when the legal relationship of women to the state and to the law was first being resolved women's subjectivity was as problematic for law as children's is today. Indeed, many of the parallels between the emancipation and consequent 'legal personing' of women and children are striking, and it is here that children's public/private violations resonate with women's history (O'Donovan, 1985). But the way in which the problematic subjectivity of women was dealt with by law was to 'fold them into the liberal batter' and to treat them in the same way as law's men: autonomous, self-interested and universal. The disadvantage women have suffered as a result of this theoretical conversion is the subject of much feminist jurisprudence.[27] Children however, cannot be made to fit so easily into the liberal legal paradigm,[28] as the public and legal anxiety and debate over Thompson and Venables's trial shows. The power of the *idea* of childhood combined with children's physical dependency remains strong, so that the paramountcy of their welfare is asserted over their rights legally. Moreover, the protection of that welfare becomes a legal, political and moral imperative. Good examples of this imperative 'in action' are the cases in which (mentally competent) children are not permitted by the law to decide that they consent to die, or even to refuse medical treatment that others feel they need.[29] How then, do we reconceive of the nature of childhood and the nature of children's subject identity when the previously taken for granted boundaries no longer make sense, but the 'easy' answer learned from women's legal personing is neither available nor desirable?

One way to deal with the confusion is to resort to the previously understood categorizations and to blame (note the moral language) the perceived causes of the disruption – for example, children and their mothers, consumerism or rights without responsibilities. We 'lash out at any potential enemy of childhood; the incompetent parent [mother] or teacher, the drug-dealer, the paedophile, the maker of the video-nasty' (Cox, 1996, p. 195) or indeed the child himself or herself. Importantly, this strategy operates to preserve and to reinforce the old categories by clarifying the exclusions from them. Thus we have constructions of childhood fortified as dependence, vulnerability and innocence[30] (personified, for example, in James and Denise Bulger: Young, 1996), and justice understood only in moral terms which confirm that innocence and the evil of those who are excluded from the category (the 'monsters' or non-children, Thompson and Venables, and their non-maternal mothers).[31]

On the other hand, we can exploit the other political possibility. We can use these moments of disruption to transcend any belief in the polarity and irreconcilability of dependence and independence, self and other, and moral and legal, and recognize that both the boundaries and the categories they create are myths. Jenks puts it well: '[c]hildren have become both the testing ground for the necessity of independence in the constitution of human subjectivity and also the symbolic refuge of the desirability of trust, dependence and care in human relations' (Jenks, 1996, p. 111). And so the way in which we construct childhood as at times the same as or at times different from adulthood and the way in which we resolve the 'test' of constituting human subjectivity do indeed provide a measure of social and legal relations generally. At this moment, when we are faced with what has been called the 'end of childhood' as we know it (Cunningham, 1995) we might be able to reformulate notions of justice which reject dichotomies previously thought to be irreducible. To reconceptualize the child subject to take some account of an alternative type of subjectivity previously attributed only to adults, without regarding such a reconceptualization as a crisis, may represent our best chance for reformulating notions of justice for children.

Autonomy, dependence and agency

> [T]he autonomy ideal encompasses two principles: the concept of individual autonomy...and the concept of respect for autonomy of others....Reciprocity is therefore inherent in the implementation of principles of autonomy....It is therefore, appropriate to conceptualise the entire structure of autonomy as one of relationship rather than independence.
>
> (Weinberg, 1995, pp. 343–4)

In this view of the autonomy usually reserved for adults, relationship rather than disconnection is presented as autonomy's framework. This view of the autonomous self contains within it an almost 'child-like' quality of dependence, and understands (adult) selfhood *as* a relation (Norrie, 1996, p. 552). This presentation recognizes that a legal subject is never abstracted and individuated, but rather always exists as a part of his or her context and relationships – even relationships based upon love rather than upon rights or exchange. Once the adult subject is understood in this way, recognizing some form of autonomy for children becomes less of a crisis. The constructed boundary between child and adult opens up.

This reformulation also attributes an agency to the subject to play a part in his or her subjectification.

> Social relations are reproduced because persons exist both as role-playing individual agents and, more fundamentally, as selves. They are created out of a language, in some ways peculiar to modern societies, of individual biography, identity and capacity for action.
>
> (Norrie, 1996, p. 552)

Childhood, like adulthood, cannot be universalized in this view, and we must then speak of childhood and adulthood in the plural. Ashe's idea of the subject's 'radical renewal' is similar; she demands an interrogation of the subject's circumstances and connections, and demands further that the subject herself or himself be allowed to present them.

Justice then requires attention to those circumstances as articulated by the subject.

This approach[32] would reveal the re-presented subject to be a product of an accumulation of understandings of different conditions in which she or he is situated, including material, social, emotional and legal conditions of both autonomy and connection, as well as of its engagement with those conditions. In moral terms, the either/or of dependence/independence may be overcome and, in legal terms, the relevance of historic or systemic conditions of advantage or disadvantage may be recognized. Finally, the dichotomy between the moral and the legal may be overcome. This is not to say that the individual rights-bearing subject would be denied an opportunity in law to speak, but is to say that the traditional terms of the subject's language, previously limited (Norrie 1996) both by law's limited conception of subjectivity and by law's normative conception of justice, would be recast. Once again, the history of the changing notions of childhood, combined with the current uncertainty of it, allows childhood to be a potentially fertile testing ground for this radical renewal of the legal subject.

I don't have a plan or a blueprint as to the process – in fact I have an ambivalent relationship with the autonomous individual and liberal legal ideas of justice for this individual. In a world where human rights matter, there *is* a degree of human dignity that autonomy and legal rights provide for people. But in my exploration of a way to bridge the gap between childhood and adulthood, and law and morality, I want to challenge the hegemony of notions of autonomy which exclude reciprocity or dependence, notions of welfare and dependence which exclude individual agency or political citizenship, and notions of boundaries which exclude the idea that those boundaries may themselves be infused with meaning and intimate connections. Justice for the related/situated subject must, therefore, be 'nuanced' (Norrie, 1996, p. 556) to take account of an individual's multiplicity of qualities as both a 'legal' and a 'moral' subject. It is the 'crisis' provoked by visible working or violent children which may provide us with an opportunity to reconceive radically what justice means for children. If it lies at the interface between the boundaries which construct their identity as distinct from adults, and so incorporates their dependence as well as their independence, their welfare as well as their rights, it may also have radical potential for justice for all.

Notes

1 I would like to acknowledge with thanks the comments of participants at the Moral Agendas for Children's Welfare workshop, Queen Mary and Westfield College Law Faculty seminar, and the Critical Legal Conference 1996, where earlier versions of this paper were presented. I also thank David Seymour, Alan Norrie, Peter Fitzpatrick and Katherine O'Donovan for their helpful comments and criticisms of many of these ideas.

2 Legal decision-making often distinguishes between the morality and the legality, or the legality and the politics of an issue. In *Re MB* [1997] 2 F.L.R. 426 at 440 the Court of Appeal had recourse to this distinction when it considered whether it was bound to take the interests of a foetus into account if these conflicted with the interests of the pregnant woman: '[A]s has so often been said, this is not a court of morals.' As a further example of the distinction, Mary-Jane Mossman (1991) discusses the spuriousness of a distinction between 'politics' and 'law'.

3 In Levinas's notion of alterity, for example, regard for and attention to the 'other' are a fundamental part of 'being': see Hand (1989). See also Norrie's (1996) use of 'critical realism' and the always situated subject.

4 This is not the same thing as justice meaning justice for the community at the expense of the individual, that which Stephen Frosh (in ch.12, this volume) describes as exemplified by the fundamentalist community which almost negates the existence of the individual for his or her own good – the good of the community. It is rather to be able to perceive the individual differently.

5 See, for example, the use of Carol Gilligan's (1982) work in legal theory, such as Bender (1988) and Frug (1992). Gilligan's work on moral development has been identified with a type of 'cultural feminism' which has been controversial among feminists.

6 For a good overview of different historical constructions of childhood, see Hendrick (1990).

7 The age or stage of development at which this occurs, is not, of course, universally agreed upon.

8 Or, perhaps, adult men. See Carol Gilligan's (1982) work.

9 A secondary relationship characterizing children's dependence and welfare is with the state.

10   Genevieve Lloyd has demonstrated how, in the seventeenth century, reason became associated with maleness; it was seen as a skill whose achievement was associated with a more adult, more masculine way of understanding and dealing with the world (Lloyd, 1984, p. 38f.). Increasingly in eighteenth-century thought, women are regarded as inhabiting a separate world of thought and feeling. This world is set in opposition to male rationality and sometimes is regarded as morally superior, but is confined to the private domestic sphere and hence acquires a special relationship with childhood (*ibid.*, pp. 57f.).
(Cox, 1996, p. 70)

11 Jenks (1996, p. 42), for example, notes that the connection of childhood and womanhood is not natural; it is a function of society's 'socio-economic requisites'.

12 Martha Fineman expresses the 'naturalization' of the relationship in broader terms which can incorporate discourses such as medicine (Rothman, 1989), social work (Lewis, 1992) and psychology (Chodorow, 1978), but recognizes their potential partiality:

> Even social or cultural institutions such as motherhood that women occupy exclusively were what I call 'colonized categories' – initially defined, controlled and given legal content by men. Male norms and male understandings [seen as universal norms and understandings] fashioned legal definitions of what constituted a family, [and] what was good mothering.....
>
> (Fineman, 1995, p. x)

Yngvesson describes it as 'naturalized' as an 'intimate, emotionally charged connection' which patriarchy manifests as outside the boundary of law, as opposed to fatherhood, grounded as it is in property rights over the child, which remains fundamentally within the law (Yngvesson, 1997, pp. 38–9).

13 I borrow this phrase from Boyd (1990).

14 See Terry Carney's ch. 4 in this volume.

15 Jenks (1996, pp. 42–3) discusses how dependence is usually associated with weakness: heroin dependency, emotional dependency, etc.

16 See also Hendrick (1990) and Donzelot (1980). There is a similar phenomenon in the history of paternalism over women's engagement with legal and social worlds – care and welfare and paternalism meant moral approval of control and disempowerment.

17 See also Cox (1996).

18 Hendrick (1990, p. 42) also suggests that it was over the issue of child labour that the qualitative difference between child and adult became accepted wisdom: 'It was, however, the issue of labour – free and unfree – (symbolized by slavery) – which gave meaning to the "fundamental categories" [child and adult].'

19 It is a breach that is not unique, however, and Hendrick (1990) maps the original construction of the boundary in the nineteenth century which resulted in the universalized conception of childhood that is again being challenged.

20 Colin Perrin 'Breath From Nowhere: Justice and Community in the Event of Human Rights', PhD thesis submitted to University of Kent at Canterbury, 1996. See Article 31, United Nations Convention on the Rights of the Child.

21 United Nations Convention on the Rights of the Child.

22 Children Act 1989 ss 1(3)(a).

23 Children Act 1989 ss 1(2)(b) and 10(8). Freeman (1992) argues for the importance of attributing rights to children, Eekelaar (1992) maintains the importance of thinking children have rights, and Archard argues that children's rights should be extended, not in an 'all or nothing' way, but in

some situations and for some children as a 'public and palpable acknowledgement of their status and worth' (Archard, 1993, p. 169).

24 In *Re B (A Minor) (Wardship: Sterilisation)* [1988] AC 199 HL, where the
court sanctioned the sterilization of a mentally impaired seventeen-year-
old woman, Lord Oliver commented at p. 211

> [t]he right to reproduce is of value only if accompanied by the ability
> to make a choice and in the instant case there is no question of the
> minor ever being able to make such a choice or indeed to appreciate
> the need to make one.

25 Cunningham (1995, pp. 160–1) describes a document drawn up by a US
child labour reformer:

> in which children 'declare ourselves to be helpless and dependent;
> that we are and of right ought to be dependent, and that we hereby
> present the appeal of our helplessness that we may be protected in the
> enjoyment of the rights of childhood'.

26 See also Bar-On (1997):

> Yet probably the most significant trait of street children is their rela-
> tionship to the public. Instead of using the street only as a channel of
> conduit between private pursuits, as most lower-and middle-class
> people do, street children spend much of their time on it and so are
> publicly visible. Their very presence thereby challenges bourgeois
> society which governs in the expectation that children will intrude as
> little as possible on the adult world, and distinguishes sharply
> between public and private.
>
> (Bar-On, 1997, p. 68)

27 In the criminal law context, see, for example, Allen (1988); in tort, see
Bender (1988); in contract, see Frug (1992).
28 In many of the same ways as women do not fit – see McDiarmid (1996).
29 See, for example, *Re W (A Minor) (Consent to Medical Treatment)* [1993] 1
F.L.R. 1.
30 Innocence here is a moral concept; law understands only a specialized
meaning of guilty or not guilty.
31 Young (1996, pp. 117–25) describes how judicial and press descriptions
of Ann Thompson and Susan Venables contrasted with that of Denise
Bulger. Bulger was constructed as a 'victim' along with her son, primarily
because she conformed to maternal convention – being with her son.
Thompson, on the other hand, was described as dry-eyed and defiant, a
troublemaker who was not with her child and not able to control her
child. Investigations into the Venables family situation as diagnosed by
Sereny's article, revealed that Susan Venables loved her son 'inappropriately', suffocating him and confusing him, and thus led to his violent
behaviour. 'These two women embody maternity as Other...based in the
confusion between their appearance as mothers and their identities (diagnosed in articles such as Sereny's) as non-maternal' (Young, 1996, p. 125).

32 This approach can be described as a feminist one, and legal method and argumentation based upon it can be described as feminist legal method. Indeed, this kind of representation of the legal subject and critique of traditional rights is a feminist approach to law and legal theory.

9   Moral agendas for psychoanalytic practice with children and families

Judith Trowell and Gillian Miles

Introduction

Psychoanalysis offers a way of understanding human beings in all their complexity including their violence, aggression, sexuality and envy. But psychoanalysis works slowly, struggles to live with uncertainty, does not make judgements, and tries to help the individual, couple or family arrive at their own thoughts, feelings and decisions. So it inevitably stands in opposition to or in conflict with elements of society that want, need, demand answers and decisions.

Psychoanalysis, unlike law, has no overt moral agenda. Psychotherapy, the therapeutic application of psychoanalysis, is non-judgemental; it requires and expects individuals to express themselves in whatever way they can, and through expression to make sense of themselves and their experiences. This is done using the relationship between the individual and the therapist as the therapeutic tool. In child protection work, the domains of child welfare and therapy intersect. Where children need protection, there may be occasions when therapists have to break the trust and confidentiality which others vest in them.

A psychoanalytic perspective highlights the irrational, it highlights uncertainty and the need at times to stay within the realm of uncertainty. Its particular emphasis is on the uniqueness of each individual; that each situation has a particular meaning for those particular individuals at that particular time. It also highlights the importance of allowing oneself to be open to the communication of others, both their conscious and unconscious communications, and to be able to bear the pain, the conflicts, and the transference and counter-transference experiences, which we explain later in this chapter. This being so, there will be dilemmas that have no easy answers.

Ideally, the therapist works with this pain and confusion, and slowly the confusion can be analysed, and the pain made manageable. But very often, uncertainty remains. How then can child protection work and the legal framework that underpins it interact with and use the knowledge arising from psychoanalytic psychotherapy? Can the therapists find a way to engage in a dialogue with the child protection system that does not damage or destroy the therapy?

Psychoanalytic psychotherapy

Working psychoanalytically with children and their families began with Freud himself and his description of the Little Hans case. Following the pioneering work of Melanie Klein and Anna Freud, the work has developed and spread, and the last fifty years has seen a vast range of innovations. The range of children seen and the kinds of difficulties which can be handled through therapy has been expanded and extended. There have been developments in individual work so that it may be either long term, open ended or brief; it may be intensive or non-intensive; it may be focused, addressing a particular difficulty, or unfocused, working across a range of problems and relationship difficulties. The work may be with individual children or with children in groups, whether sibling groups, open groups, groups for children with a specific issue or with families.

Where the children are seen separately, the parents, parent or carers are seen for parallel work. This work may be supportive to help the parent bring the child and manage practical issues. It may be psychotherapeutic to help parents explore the issues for themselves and their family that link with the child's problems and the part played by the family dynamics of all its members; or, alternatively, it may be psychotherapy for the parent in his or her own right. Carers/parents may be seen individually or as a couple, as dealing with marital issues frequently forms part of the work.

At the same time as the growth and development of psychoanalytic or psychoanalytically informed work with children and families, there has been a fundamental shift in social attitudes, firstly towards women, and latterly in regard to children, which has had fundamental implications for psychoanalytic practice. Freud working with troubled Little Hans, saw and discussed the problems only with the father; he did not himself see mother or little Hans or the family; the discussions were with father and the therapy was conducted by father. This may seem shocking to us now but, within the context of Viennese society at that time, it represented a pioneering piece of work. After all, Freud did listen and take seriously what his female patients said to him, just as he took seriously what Little Hans said and recognized the significance of his behaviour.

What does psychoanalytic work with children and families involve?

The core of psychoanalytic theory is based on the belief that there is an unconscious. According to this belief, the unconscious arises both from within the individual and from without. From birth (or perhaps prior to birth), the baby is managing sensations and feelings that arise both inside the body and impact on the body from outside (Freud, 1933). Gradually, these sensations and feelings are integrated and sense is made of them (Winnicott, [1962] 1976). Crucial in this process is the mother, the primary carer who responds to the baby with intuition and empathy derived from her capacity for projective identification (Bion, 1962). Verbally, and non-verbally, the mother communicates to the baby that these sensations and feelings can be felt both as emotions – anger, hurt, pain, delight, love, pleasure – and can also be thought about, given names and expressed symbolically through words. Hence the development of language, play, knowledge and thinking (Klein, [1921] [1928] 1975).

Alongside the development of the conscious, many sensations, thoughts and feelings remain unconscious, that is, they are not accessible to the individual. Individuals take in a whole range of sensations, feelings, experiences, relationships, that originate in the external world. Many of these thoughts and feelings remain conscious, but they may also become part of the unconscious, joining with the individual's own internal experiences to make the internal world. This process is unique to each person, although there are common characteristics.

The internal world has in it internal objects – that is, key relationship figures (Fairbairn, 1954, Winnicott, [1945] 1958; Klein, [1935] 1975). For example, the mother as internal object, may comprise what the mother actually is and does, the conscious memory of how mother was, together with the unconscious wishes, longing, frustrations that occurred both early on and subsequently in relation to the mother. This internal object mother together with all the other internal objects are in a dynamic relationship in the internal world, which exists simultaneously with occurrences in the external world. The state of the internal world has a considerable effect on how the individual reacts in the present, in the external world.

Psychoanalytic work is based on the view that problems can be understood in terms of conflicts. These conflicts are both in the external world, but more importantly, can originate in the internal world, or at the boundary between these two worlds. Unresolved issues in the internal world, whether they arise from unconscious fantasies that have not been processed, or from a combination of external past or present events and these unconscious fantasies, give rise to the symptoms, problems and difficulties that psychoanalytic work tries to address. This work is carried out by using the relationship with the therapist in the here and now as a tool. During interviews, the therapist tries to identify from conversation or play what is being communicated. These verbal and non-verbal communications are enriched and enlightened by the unconscious communications of transference and counter-transference. 'Transference' is the term used to describe the feelings and responses to the therapist that the patient brings to the therapy arising from both their previous experience with others but also their longings and fears that have arisen from actual relationships, and also from fantasies in their own internal world. Counter-transference is used to describe the thoughts and feelings that arise in the therapist in response to the patient's 'transference'. This response in the therapist needs careful monitoring, as the reaction may be due to the therapist's own difficulties. Very often, however, counter-transference can be of help to a well-trained therapist as the 'counter-transference' can provide a means of understanding what is occurring within the relationship in the room that is not being explicitly expressed. Both what the person says, does and conveys, and what is not said, but is experienced by the therapist, is used as a means of understanding the child, adult or family. The therapeutic relationship is, therefore, the key therapeutic tool, and within this relationship conflictual thoughts and feelings can be experienced and understood.

Within this analytic way of thinking, concepts such as defences or defence mechanisms, containment, projective identification and introjection are used to explain what occurs, as well as ideas about the capacity to symbolize, think, make links and tolerate uncertainty. Alongside these hypotheses about the complexity of human beings, there are also views about a developmental process that explains emotional development, and the development of sexuality and morality in the individual.

Psychoanalytic work struggles with the range of human experience, mental and emotional, mental illness, life events, the impact of physical illness, relationship problems, offending behaviour, trauma, deprivation, by working with confusion, turmoil, conflicts and fantasies, holding in mind that the physical body must also be given importance at all times.

The impact of social changes on psychoanalytic work

Psychotherapists are inevitably influenced by the context in which they work. In England and Wales, the introduction of the Children Act 1989, in October 1991, and the ratification by the British Government of the United Nations Convention on the Rights of the Child, in December 1991, have changed the framework within which therapy operates. Children now have a right to have their needs recognized and met. They also have the right to be protected, to be given choices, and to have their own views taken seriously.

These changes arose from an acknowledgement that children are individuals who deserve to be treated with respect and to be taken seriously. There is an ongoing debate about what constitutes children's rights and whether children should have rights without the accompanying responsibilities. But what has been crucial for psychotherapeutic purposes has been the recognition that children have their own wishes, thoughts and feelings, and that these need to be heard and given consideration even if adults do not agree with what the child wants. It is now widely accepted that children need, and should be given, an explanation so they can see that their views were heard, even if they cannot be acted on at that time.

All of this, however, raises moral dilemmas for psychotherapists working with children. What should a therapist do if a child talks in therapy about a home situation that could be indicative of abuse, but begs the therapist to promise not to tell anyone? The child does not want the family involved but the therapist's concerns are such that he or she may be required to break the child's trust and inform a child protection agency. If this occurs, the therapist might be instrumental in bringing about the very thing that the child dreads. Psychotherapists, therefore, are now in a position that may involve setting the child's wishes against his or her interests and setting the child against the parents. This occurs within the context of a legal and normative framework that appears to give more weight than in the past to the wishes and views of children but that, when these laws and norms are translated into practice, in fact, gives more weight to the wishes and needs of parents.

When issues of protection are involved, the law requires therapists to use their clinical judgement only up to a certain point and then blames them when decisions retrospectively are seen to be wrong. This leaves them in a moral dilemma – when should they wait and try to explore further, when should they speak out? They have to ask themselves, 'Whom are we protecting, the child or the child's parents?'

Particular moral issues

Therapists and child protection

As indicated, the success of psychoanalysis and psychotherapy depends on the therapists' use of themselves as a receptor, a tool that identifies processes, makes sense of conflicts and tries to understand problems from this perspective. This means the therapist's training, supervision and own personality and emotional agendas are crucial. The training involves careful selection of suitable individuals who are then taught theory, child development and a range of skills, and provided with supervised experience. The training also insists that the therapist's own unresolved emotional issues have been addressed and that the therapist is aware when their own current or past emotions and conflicts interfere with the work, and what should be done if this occurs. Therapists generally need some ongoing consultation or supervision to help them sustain the ethical practice they have been taught; that is, to maintain their professional relationship at all times, not using patients for their own gratification, and keeping their patients' best interests central to the work.

Given that most therapy at times involves intense feelings – rage, hate, need, longing for love, and sexual feelings – there is a particular moral dilemma. Therapists may feel it is cruel to deny patients gratification. This can culminate in a moral crisis when inappropriate anger, physical contact, physical abuse or sexual contact occurs. How do therapists know what is right or wrong? They can only know what are the prevailing moral standards in the country where they work and in the training establishment where they were trained. Different cultures and different ethnic groups may place differing emphases on what is expected of children, young people and their families. The task of the therapist, as far as possible, is to assist their patients to resolve their conflicts and distress from earlier experiences or arising in their internal world so that they have the freedom to develop their potential and to make choices less hindered by old traumas and emotional pain or confusion. Child protection work can conflict with this therapeutic work and 'bad' therapy may result.

As we have previously stated, the legal system requires certainty, and therapy, in contrast, is predicated on the ability to live with uncertainty and ambiguity. Child protection decisions also require clarity. If during the course of treatment it appears that the child may have been abused, the therapist may need to change his or her therapeutic way of working according to the need to question and seek answers, to try and ascertain the facts, or at least get sufficient evidence to decide whether to alert the child protection agencies. It may not be possible subsequently to restore the therapeutic alliance and resume the therapeutic work.

Bad training may not prepare therapists adequately for the rigour and demands of the work. Training that does not require therapists to have their own therapy leaves their trainees vulnerable to unexpected emotional reactions which they are likely to find difficult to control or of which they may not even be aware when they occur with the patient. Bad training can also teach theory and skills without ensuring the personal development needed to be able to weigh complex situations in the balance and arrive at sound decisions for the patients, such as when to stay silent and when to speak out.

The imbalance in power between therapist and patient, and the patient's confusion and need leaves them vulnerable not only to gross exploitation, but also either to the more subtle over-involvement or holding-on that can occur, or to precipitate termination of treatment when the therapist feels overwhelmed. It can be very easy to explain such decisions in terms of the patients' resistance or with reference to the counter-transference rather than to face what has really been going on between therapist and patient.

Working with children is particularly difficult, given the need for a much more active technique. Children need to go to the toilet, they run, climb all over the furniture, play dangerously, climb on laps, hit, kick, bite and spit. Maintaining a therapeutic stance in such situations is very challenging and the dilemmas facing the therapist are little acknowledged. One such is the issue of restraint and coercion, which for the therapist is a profound moral dilemma. Is it ever appropriate and if so, what form should it take? If children or young people do not wish to participate in the therapeutic work, then the dilemma is stark. Should they be coerced, in the hope that once begun they will appreciate the benefit of therapy, or should they be allowed to decline treatment? If they consistently refuse to attend or enter the room despite explanations and encouragement from parents, carers and therapist, in reality, little can be done. If parents or carers are uncertain about the help or silently hostile, it may not be possible to engage the parents in helping the child to feel less fearful and anxious. Some young people are able to attend and engage in work in spite of parental hostility but this does need care and thought as it raises issues of loyalty and how to retain parental support which is crucial to the success of the therapy.

If patients attempt to injure themselves or the therapist, or damage objects in the room, restraint may be needed, particularly if the attacks are such that serious injury may result. Once the safety of the child and the therapist has been ensured, the therapist still needs to manage his or her own feelings of fear and the human wish to retaliate if hurt. If an individual child or young person has needed to be restrained, it is important to record it and share the information with the parents or carer. Where there might be bruising or the child removes clothes and engages in socially unacceptable sexual behaviour, the therapist has to struggle with restraining the child, whilst not rejecting him or her. How to manage future therapy sessions will need considerable thought. The risks for the child and therapist also need thought; to go on is difficult, to stop may be damaging. The dilemma for the therapist is whether to continue, to prevent the child from experiencing rejection, nevertheless facing the risk of being accused of engaging in unacceptable physical contact.

If families are sent to the clinic by the courts or Social Services and they themselves do not want to be there, see no reason to be there, and do not consider that they need any therapeutic help, the therapist is obliged to decide whether or not to try and impose therapy. It may be that, in spite of their reluctance, as the therapeutic work progresses, the parents or children begin to understand and change, and then choose to co-operate. Then again, they may not. Many therapists refuse to work in this way, but some will offer a trial period. This dilemma reflects the contrasting attitudes of therapy and the law.

Some families forced to come may decide they have to comply, and so appear to co-operate after initial resistance. Deceit is not always easy to detect and so bad therapy may be carried out, because it is based on lies. Anti-therapeutic therapy can also occur (Furniss, 1991). This happens when an abused child is brought for treatment and the family appears to be co-operative, but in reality the abuse is continuing and the therapy is based on falsehood. The parents' intention is here not to assist the child's recovery but to divert attention away from what is going on covertly. It is bad therapy in that the therapist has not ensured that those responsible for the child's safety have done what was required. The child is left in a damaging situation believing the therapist is colluding with the abuse by continuing to work alongside it.

Confidentiality

Parents frequently find it very difficult not to know what is occurring during the therapy with their child. This is not surprising, but the therapeutic work is predicated on the child being free to say whatever he or she is thinking or feeling without any judgements being made. Whatever emerges can be thought about and accepted as part of the work. As they struggle with their feelings, children are often worried that their parents will be told. However, there are some basic concerns which need to be shared with parents and the therapist will need to exercise judgement as to what, if anything, to say and how not to betray the child's trust.

As concern over child abuse has increased, confidentiality has become an even greater moral dilemma, particularly in cases where abuse was not originally suspected. It may be good for the therapy to keep confidentiality but bad for protection of the child in cases where abuse continues to occur. When children start to share information that raises concerns, therapists have to record the sessions very carefully, and need to keep a balance between respecting the child's trust and the need to keep the child safe. Frequently, the basis of concern is vague – is the child talking about a dream, or a wish or longing, or is the child hinting at something that has really happened? Each case needs to be considered separately and the level of anxiety monitored. When the information from children is both consistent and of major concern, the child should be informed that confidentiality will be broken and given an explanation as to why this has to happen. Work will then need to take place to preserve the therapeutic alliance.

Work with the parent(s) or carer(s) can also raise child protection concerns directly or indirectly. The work needs to continue while, at the same time, the parent should be encouraged to contact Social Services. If this does not happen, the workers have to explain why Social Services will be informed against the wishes of the parent. Making this decision can present the workers with a moral dilemma, since it involves not only the child's best interest, but also the workers' anxiety about whether or not the information should be passed on, and the workers' need to protect themselves professionally.

Reporting abuse has become a dilemma for therapists because of anxiety about the effect on the 'therapeutic relationship'. It is felt to be a betrayal of trust and yet it is also recognized that even where the child or parent becomes angry or subsequently denies the information, it is important to take these concerns seriously. The therapist's decision is difficult in that it cuts across the rules and boundaries of the therapeutic relationship. It may be tempting for the therapist to avoid the issue.

Consent

In the UK the issues presented by consent have had to be rethought, after the introduction of the Patient's Charter (Department of Health and Social Services, 1991b). Can both parents and children give consent to psychoanalytic treatment for the child? They can be offered help for their problems and the treatment may be described in advance, but until they experience the therapy, it is difficult for either of them to give fully informed consent.

Many therapists find managing the need to obtain consent difficult, seeing it as a potential intrusion into the development of the therapeutic process. It is possible to talk about the process of making conflicts conscious and offering help to resolve these conflicts so that choices and decision-making become more objective, but such accounts do not convey the pain, struggle and distress of the therapy. Normally, parental consent is required and the children are informed. Even where children do give their express agreement, it is unlikely that they really understand what is involved.

Consent arises again as an issue with children when they wish to stop the therapy or when child protection issues emerge. Some children want to stop because they find therapy is not right for them. They are correct in thinking that they cannot benefit from this type of intervention. But children may also want to stop if they are working with the therapist on particularly painful issues, such as the effect of a parent dying, abuse, the move to another foster placement or the breakdown of a previous fostering. It is difficult to know when it is right to stop therapy. A decision has to be made. Is the child not psychologically ready to work? Should he or she, on the other hand, be brought to a realization that, despite the protests, the work should continue, because the therapy has reached a critical but very painful point? Occasionally, consent comes from elsewhere – parents, social worker, or sometimes the courts, who ask for or order that work be done. Some therapists do not feel able to work in such circumstances. Others try to see the longer term benefits for the child and continue to offer therapy and engage the child.

Giving evidence in court

Many therapists will not attend court. They feel that to do so breaks the therapeutic relationship. This is right to some extent, and often it is preferable if another member of the team who is not doing the direct work, should attend court instead. The professional who goes to court takes the moral decision that what has emerged gives rise to a cause for concern about the child's welfare, and leaves the therapist to continue the therapeutic work. The situation is different if the case and the work were a 'court' case from the start. Then the child, the carers/parents and the professionals are aware throughout that there will be a hearing.

Where cases that start as clinical cases become court cases, there can be further dilemmas. The therapist may be called, records and notes may be subpoenaed. Is the psychoanalytic discourse appropriate in court? The play, the dreams, the free association, the transference and counter-transference are not hard facts; rather they are a means, a way, to understand what the conflict, the problem, was about, in order to work further on it within therapy. From this, one might be able to comment on the mental state of the individual and have a view about events, but this form of information is not 'evidence', or legal facts.

Finding a way to use the psychoanalytic perspective, the understanding arrived at in this way is not easy and takes time and skill. There is an innate tension between a legal discourse and a psychoanalytic discourse. Evidence, 'the facts', are vital to make decisions in court. The psychoanalytic discourse values uncertainty, not knowing, and slow thoughtful exploration, and there are times when attempts to introduce the content of therapy sessions into court discussions can be damaging, distorting the material as well as betraying the child (King and Trowell, 1992). Psychotherapy is a resource to which individuals may turn for help. Difficult moral issues arise when it is used to find definite answers or with the spoken or unspoken aim of turning troubled individuals into socially acceptable citizens.

Parenting and cultural issues

Psychoanalysis offers views on the emerging relationship between children and their parents. For example, the Oedipal conflict and the role of father and mother in the children's internal world as well as the external world is seen as crucial. There is also a view about certain facts that children need to know. These may be summarized as:

- the life span
- birth, death
- generational differences (children, parents, grandparents)
- physical differences – male and female (Kyrle, 1932).

These ideas may cause conflicts and dilemmas in relation to changes in society that rightly demand respect and equality for each individual. How do psychoanalysts think, when working with children and families, about single parents, same-sex parents, cross-generational relationships and the differing child-rearing practices in the many cultures that make up our society? Most therapists come from a narrow class, cultural and racial background, and their body of theory was developed by intellectuals who also came from this narrow background.

Psychoanalytic child development sees the primary carer (usually mother) as crucial. From this perspective, children who have had a number of primary and secondary carers may feel misunderstood, undervalued, denigrated. This is particularly so if there are skin colour differences. Psychoanalytic ideas have been seen as Eurocentric. The developing understanding of attachment theory means that today we have a better understanding of how key relationships evolve for all children (Bowlby, 1988). In addition, the development of sexual identity is being explored, and psychoanalysts now recognize the importance of the development of the internal world with its internal object relations in parallel but separate from the external world (Klein, [1945] 1975). In addition, therapists have their own personal views on these matters, which inevitably emerge in the course of their work with children, despite all their attempts to suppress them.

Disability can also present problems for therapists. Parents with a physical disability or a learning disability are frequently seen in terms of the disability first, rather than as a person who has a disability. There is much to learn about how parenting is affected and what is good enough. Very often adults with a disability are seen as incapable of parenting, and judgements are made without really evaluating the individual. Perhaps the most important issue is how able the parent is to be available emotionally for the child, to 'contain' them so that they feel valued and understood. The practical arrangements should be secondary but, of course, resources are such that this is not the case. It is much easier to make an impersonal decision on the basis of the disability. However, unless the disturbance is gross, such as in the case of a psychotic mother who involves the child in her hallucinations and delusions or a learning disabled parent who cannot manage daily life, most children are able to develop satisfactorily with a parent who has a disability. Therapists, when asked for their opinion, frequently assume that serious disability precludes parenting and so avoid the problems of having to weigh up the possibilities carefully and arrive at a considered decision.

Breaking up families

Where there are issues of child protection or inadequate parenting, there is a dilemma for psychoanalytic workers in facing the break-up of families. Divorce, where the family is split up by the adults, is less of a dilemma although equally distressing. The real moral dilemma for the therapist arises when they conclude that they need to initiate an action that could lead to the break-up of a family. When working closely with children and their families, it can become too painful for therapists even to consider suggesting that the family needs to split up or the child be removed.

In psychoanalytic terms, object relations and attachments are established very early and from then on the key individuals are important in the child's life. Knowing this can lead to endless attempts to work for change, even though the possibility of the adult changing in time to avoid too much damage to the child is virtually impossible.

Balancing the needs of the child, the wishes of the child, and the capacities and needs of parents is acutely distressing. More so because a psychoanalytic therapist knows that it is not possible for children to be removed, placed in another family and have a fresh start, cutting off awareness of the past. Children's internal object relationships will go with them and influence their ongoing relationships. We now see many children who were fostered or adopted seeking out their family of origin in order to understand themselves, and this phenomenon links closely with the psychoanalytic view. So there is a real dilemma here. Can children have the choice to stay with their parents, or should they be removed against their wishes? And what role should the psychoanalytic therapist take?

Specific conditions

Contraceptives, anorexia and bulimia, suicide attempts and mental illness all present problems and raise moral dilemmas. In situations involving patients who are chronologically adolescent, and so seen as capable of making their own decisions, the psychoanalytic dilemma can be acute. It may be apparent in therapy that the individual is still very much younger psychically, or there may be many unconscious confusions and fantasies that are preoccupying the individual's mind. Death may be seen by the patient as a way of taking revenge or joining a loved one. Death may have all sorts of meanings and offer all kinds of fantasies, including the possibility that death itself may not be permanent. How actively should a therapist intervene to prevent a suicide? Does the young person have the right to choose life or death?

Birth and babies may also be a source of confusion. In the mind of the patient, babies may be conceived orally, made up of faeces, produced by the individual alone; food and its ingestion may be seen as a way of producing a baby. In this confused internal state, should a young person, intent on having sexual intercourse, be encouraged to seek contraceptive advice? Does the therapist accept the fact that the patient is physically capable of sexual intercourse despite emotional immaturity and encourage the use of precautions, or does he or she try to address the emotional issues?

So issues about contraception, suicide attempts and eating disorders, all to do with life and death, may have many more unconscious meanings than the apparent external reality. There is frequently a dilemma about how to think about these issues and the patient's decision-making capacity when the unconscious may be in turmoil, but the external calm and rational. There is no answer except to explore each case individually, but this does not fit with the desire for a social order ruled by guidelines and procedures.

The treatment of mental illness presents other problems and moral decisions to be made by the therapist. A depressed young person or a person with a discrete psychotic or delusional system may function in some settings. A psychoanalytic practitioner may be acutely aware of the disturbance, but uncertain when to insist on treatment against the individual's will. There is a dilemma: does the therapist, who is aware of the unconscious conflicts and the relief that could be achieved in therapy, accept that the young person has the right to live his or her own life, and refuse treatment? Should the therapist continue to accept this where the outcome is likely to be that young person's suicide or does the therapist take on the task of instigating active treatment to keep a patient alive so that treatment can continue?

So called 'false memory syndrome' also merits some thought as a specific condition. Some children have been abused but have 'forgotten' about it. During their therapy, memories may surface and can be discussed and understood. In the case of some children, the therapist may be aware of the possibility of past abuse, but throughout the therapy both therapist and child remain uncertain whether it happened or not. In the case of other children, memories of abusive experiences may emerge during the therapy when no-one had previously suspected that abuse had occurred. Children may, during therapy, become convinced they were abused. Can the therapist determine whether abuse did in fact occur? Should therapists be involved in this issue? They are thrown into a dilemma: they want to be sensitive to and supportive of their patient, but they can easily become convinced themselves that abuse has occurred, rather than stay with the uncertainty and try to help their patient tolerate this 'not knowing'. False memory syndrome may exist, it may be that the 'remembered' abuse did not actually occur. For some the memory may be of real abuse, but the therapist who becomes part of any legal battle providing corroboration of abuse needs to consider very carefully the dangers involved in translating psychoanalytic psychotherapeutic knowledge into factual knowledge.

Moral development

Psychoanalytic theory has a particular view of moral development, seeing the emergence of the 'conscience' and the ideal to be aimed for (ego ideal) as a part of evolution that crucially depends on the child's carers as well as on societal norms. Where patients are in an environment which maintains a developed sense of morality, the child is likely to develop an inner sense of their own personal morality in the process of their emotional and psychological development. If this sense of morality is lacking, is it seen as part of the therapist's work to impart a sense of morality? Small children usually have a clear sense of right and wrong, fair and unfair. Initially, it depends on being found out or not, and on ownership (having is owning). But gradually such values evolve through thinking about the impact on the wronged and also through the general development of concern, guilt and the wish to make reparation. Where the child's moral development has been deficient or absent, therapists tend to convey their own views, standards, expectations. The ways in which individuals behave and treat others is part of the work of therapy and, inevitably, during the course of that therapy, the therapist is bound to reveal something of his or her own moral views. It is not always easy or clear to distinguish which aspects of such views arise from white European culture, which aspects from psychoanalytic ideas? It is also unclear how cultures and religions with different moral codes find a place. This issue is seldom addressed and is worth further study (see Frosh, Chapter 12, this volume).

Conclusion

It does seem that all the intellectual debate and all the struggles and arguments over the minutiae of the precise meaning and use of words will not help to solve the problems that we have identified. There is also a danger that psychoanalytic practitioners may become so immersed in their work that they are unable or unwilling to look up and see the external world, preferring the internal world in which they operate. The issue would seem to be whether the moral dilemmas which the external world imposes can be recognized within the therapeutic experience, and whether they can be acknowledged and discussed, so that therapists, the children and their families, can be clear what the dilemmas are and how they are being addressed.

10 With justice in mind

Complexity, child welfare and the law

Andrew Cooper

Justice, relationships and society

The purpose of this chapter is to contribute to our thinking about the nature of justice for children and their families. In particular, I want to explore how the formal institutions we have created to respond to situations of known or suspected child abuse and family disruption do or don't 'do justice' to children's experience and that of their families. In Britain, and in most West European countries these institutions are significantly related to, derived from, or intended to act as alternatives to judicial ones. What kind of social and professional activity 'child protection and welfare' is taken to be, and to which recognized social domain it should be primarily referred, has long been a contested matter – for example in the well-worn debate between 'welfare' and 'justice' models of intervention. My contention is that a close examination of the character of these institutions, and the complex social and psychological functions they perform, particularly when undertaken from the perspective of children, abusers and the nature of abusive relationships, reveals basic confusions about their social purposes. This is because we have constructed or adapted them on the basis of a set of pre-existing categories, both with respect to what sort of occurrence child abuse is, and how society should respond to it. However, I argue that there is now a need to think completely new thoughts about these questions, and that we have gathered enough understanding to attempt this task.

The main objective of this chapter is to develop a philosophical line of thought which argues for the moral significance of a particular way of understanding child abuse and family dysfunction. This understanding is firmly linked to questions about the social organization of our responses to these problems. The argument draws on both research findings about the organization of child protection systems in Europe, and first- and second-hand clinical material involving children and adults. However, this clinical material is mainly used as a source for developing the philosophical argument, and is not intended to represent a comprehensive survey of the implications of such work for the relationship between child abuse, psychotherapy and judicial intervention. How clinicians working with children and families negotiate the difficult boundary between the psychotherapeutic and legal domains, and the ways in which the law may become a dimension of the treatment situation, are the subject of Roger Kennedy's book, *Child Abuse, Psychotherapy and the Law* (1997). It is based on lengthy experience of work with families at the Cassel Hospital, and the interested reader will find it a rich source of discussion about the complexities of this area, approached primarily through a clinician's preoccupations.

To some degree, an examination of the variety of institutions and practices which different (but in the global scheme actually rather similar) societies have created to respond to children abused or at risk, itself reveals a startling lack of consensus about these questions. In effect, this variety of institutional forms represents a range of answers to the question 'Why and how do we want to protect children?' The abuse of children, within or without their family of origin, is a phenomenon which cannot be fully represented in a single discourse or by a single person – it is at once a story of individual suffering and psychic damage; of social transgression and legal guilt; of fractured but usually not completely severed intimate relationships; of exploitation and the creation of closed worlds governed by secrets and lies; of the vulnerability of the powerless to exploitation by the powerful (and vice versa, although this is less often understood); and, not least, the corruption of the moral universe of the family. There is, in my view, no way of singling out one of these perspectives as privileged, as the only right and proper basis for our primary mode of social, legal or therapeutic response to abuse. However, each society has, usually more by accident than design, tended to privilege some particular form of response, and this is manifest in the character of its central institutions dedicated to child welfare.

One way of assessing or evaluating a society's stance towards the problem of child abuse and protection, is to ask 'How many ways of telling and understanding the story of abuse are facilitated by its official modes of response?' Or perhaps, 'How connected to one another are different versions of the story allowed to become or remain?' These are not abstract or indulgent questions. A central feature of the operation of the child protection system in England and Wales (and Scotland to a significant extent) in recent decades, has been the dominance of 'binary', either/or modes of thinking and intervention in the lives of children and their families; societal pressures and professional anxieties have given rise to official imperatives to decide that children are abused or not abused, protected or not protected, permanently placed or 'drifting', subject to good outcomes or bad, and so on. These are false certainties, and specious distinctions. Children who suffer in the particular ways we refer to as 'abuse' are typically placed in impossible psychological predicaments, and this is as true for those we think of as primarily 'physically abused' as it is for those who suffer sexual abuse. The most extreme and well-documented of these predicaments may be the guilty secrecy which pervades the incestuous relationship, but every practitioner can attest to the genuine ambivalence and fear which may attend a young child's disclosure of routine physical abuse.

We now understand that most children who are the objects of abuse or the victims of parental conflict and separation want two things – for the abuse or uncertainty to stop, and to stay with their families, or very close to them. But we can only be sure 'what children want' if we create conditions under which children are able to find out what they think about their own predicaments, and this is not something which courts have been designed to facilitate. However, when we do make this possible, we are also likely to find that the outcome is not anything which can be easily handled by courts working in an adversarial mode, and possibly not by any kind of court. More inclusion of children's views about their own situations is as likely to increase the complexity and uncertainty of decision-making as it is to decrease it. I would propose that 'binary' (either/or) modes of thinking, intervention, and decision-making in institutional life are by themselves inimical to the project of achieving adequate justice or 'good outcomes' for children. However, the difficulty and the challenge with which we are faced is that children's predicaments require decisions to be made, and decisions do always take a binary form.

Our formal response to such situations ideally requires us to think and act in at least three interrelated dimensions:

- By creating the conditions in which children can tell their story, or recover the *ability* to tell their story, and be understood, so that their view of their own predicament can be communicated effectively by them (or by an interlocutor) to the court or those with decision-making powers.
- By having at our disposal sufficient authority, practical options or psychological leverage to begin to prevent further abuse, including

the 'abuse' arising from repeated and long-term indecision and uncertainty in family conflicts.

- By having at our disposal sufficient authority, practical options or psychological leverage to set in train a process of change or better management of relationships, which will maintain optimal connection between family members under highly unpropitious circumstances.

Thus, there is a psychological and intra-psychic dimension, an inter-personal dimension and a social dimension to this project. Traditionally, these different dimensions have been reflected in the separate institutional responsibilities and activities of, respectively, psychotherapists, the courts and social workers. It is, of course, well recognized that these domains and the activities of professionals within them overlap, as well as being a source of institutional tension, inter-professional rivalry and struggle for power. Michael King and his colleagues (King and Piper, 1995; King and Trowell, 1992) have examined the problems of rival epistemologies which inform and construct different dimensions of welfare practice, and the practical consequences of the incommensurability of different professional world-views for the ideal of collaboration around a common task, as well as the trend towards the eclipse of one (the clinical or welfare) by another (the forensic or legal).

However, across this spectrum from the intra-psychic to the social, the question of re-establishing authority in places where there has been a breakdown of authority, is ubiquitous. But once again, as the study of institutional forms in different societies reveals, social, psychological, and legal authority can be brought into more or less connection with one another according to how the institutions in question conduct themselves. What is clearest is that the use of authority in response to child and family welfare problems is almost never absolute. Rather, different degrees of *semi-compulsion* are the norm in the effort to establish or re-establish psychological, social or legal order. The significance of this lies in recognizing that authority is always deployed in the context of social relationships, and that whereas some countries use extremely formal and legalized mechanisms which disguise or reify this relational element, others use more informal, dialogic, and nego-tiative methods in pursuit of the same ends. In Britain there has been an unfortunate evolution towards denying that authority is inevitably inscribed in the non-legal sphere and that it may be deployed to posi-tive social and psychological ends by professionals working with families and children. As a consequence, judicial authority itself has also tended to become reinforced by professionals as something 'external', rather than integral to the total situation of the child and family, in which professionals are also actors.

Thus far, then, I am proposing that:

- An understanding of child and family welfare problems cannot be referred to any single intellectual category or institutional domain, and always potentially involves intra-psychic, interpersonal and socio-legal considerations. These perspectives generate different 'stories' or discursively located narratives.
- A review of different countries' social and institutional arrangements for responding to child abuse and welfare problems reveals that there is no universal model or concept of justice at work in this sphere. While they may have features in common, the key institutions, practices and principles by which they operate are unique products of unique configurations of historical, cultural, political and professional factors.
- In the course of responding or intervening, some countries' systems and institutions allow more interplay between different (psychological, interpersonal, social) dimensions of the total situation, than do others.
- The use of authority in relation to perceived transgressions of social or familial norms is always implicit or explicit in the social response (however 'informal') to child abuse or child welfare problems. Thus, crucially, different levels or articulations of authority are brought into more or less connection through different institutional forms and system responses.

The above suggests that the key institutions of child welfare, including the courts, while they may explicitly take their primary task to be 'the protection of children' or the 'safeguarding of family welfare' or something similar, are important sites of *social reproduction*. On the assumption that one may most easily find evidence of a society's basic assumptions about its own conceptions of social order where it intervenes to respond to transgressions of this order, child welfare institutions are a case in point. Because, to put it rather simply, child welfare and protection are about how people should and should not treat one another in rather basic ways, important aspects of the society's *moral order* are also revealed in these entities. Because we find that different countries deploy very different means of responding to these instances of social and moral transgression, and of encouraging a restoration of order, we may discern something of how particular societies conceive the *nature of social and moral order and the conditions of its perpetuation*; for example, what balance of persuasion, negotiation, coercion or supervision is thought necessary or socially healthy in relation to its citizens in particular circumstances. The more inclusive view of child welfare institutions and practices proposed here suggests that their ultimate social purpose can be conceived in much wider terms than simply that of 'protecting children', as something more like 'ensuring minimally damaged future citizens'. For children are future citizens, and the manner in which they are or are not enabled to be actors in the effort to ameliorate their own adversity is a significant register of how a society believes its own better aspects are to be reproduced or preserved.

Complexity, particularity and universality – the dilemmas of justice

One objective of this chapter is to argue that we do not know what we mean by the concept of 'child protection', largely because we are constrained in our thinking *by* traditional categories such as 'justice', 'welfare' or 'therapy', notwithstanding the now well-documented tensions between them. Second, I argue that we do have available the intellectual equipment and research evidence to enable us to 'think new thoughts' in this area, and here I look to the work of Michael Walzer and John Gray among others. Third, because child abuse and protection demands that we think and act across the traditional boundaries which have demarcated the theoretical and practical domains of intra-psychic, interpersonal and social worlds, we cannot avoid engagement with increased complexity and methodological 'particularity' in our thinking and practice. I aim to show how this increased complexity might be coherently grasped in just one dimension – the nature of justice in its application to children and family life. Fourth, I posit that the diversity of actually existing forms of child protection and welfare systems and institutions in historically closely related societies alerts us to the fact of particularity on a different dimension – laterally (as it were) across historical time and geographical space rather than vertically through intra-psychic, micro- and macro-social space.

The argument that particularity – the derivation of judicial norms and practices from local rather than universal conditions and principles – not only exists in the realm of judicial and welfare systems, but *ought* to exist, if it is to be adequate (do justice) to the nature of the human situations to which it responds, runs counter to traditional

'universalist' conceptions of justice and welfare. The charge of ethical
and cultural relativism follows quickly after. My response to this is to
draw upon recent thinking about ideas of 'complex fairness' (Gray,
1996) and 'complex equality' (Walzer, 1983). Complexity, and its close
relative 'difference' are the uncomfortable facts of social and personal
life, to which late modernity has increasingly exposed us. One response
to this state of affairs, represented by an 'anything goes' postmodernity,
has been to celebrate our liberation from the oppressive task of
searching for some reliable ground of moral and social conduct. If this
will not do, as it clearly will not, since we must in any particular situation find ways of settling disputed moral questions such as 'What are
the limits of acceptable behaviour by these adults towards these children?', these methods must take account *both* of particularity *and* of the
presence of some socially agreed criteria for the settlement of such
disputes; however, the idea of socially agreed criteria does not in any
way imply absolute universality or timelessness. Awareness of different
and changing judicial principles and practices across time and space
should not be taken as evidence of the failure of these to conform to, or
apply, universal principles; rather they *reveal* the true nature of justice
as a social phenomenon, subject to change and alteration as a result of
social contest and debate. From here it is a short step to a conception
of specific judicial processes as deliberative or dialogic, as exercises in
structured *negotiation* within particular culturally and historically
specific circumstances, rather than the stern, scientific and alienated
application of the majesty of the law to the particular case. And
indeed, this is a conception of justice which may be found in some
European countries' children's courts. *Justice negocié* is how the work of
the French Children's Judge has sometimes been characterized
(Garapon, 1989).

What, if anything, can be said to safeguard such processes and
procedures as *justice*, rather than the arbitrary institutionalization of
particular vested social interests in a place which happens to be called a
court? My contention is that across the diversity of institutional forms
which we find in the realm of child and family justice and welfare it is
possible to answer this question by reference to the presence or absence
of something called judicial thinking or reasoning. Unquestionably,
the premises from which a French Children's Judge begins her or his
deliberations about a case, and the conclusions she or he reaches, are
often different from those which would pertain in a similar case in
England; but, in between, something recognizably the same is occurring in both countries. What kind of material (evidence, opinion,
professional assessment, testimony) is presented in what form (written

deposition, oral statement, video recording, children's drawings), according to what procedures with what aims (cross-examination, dialogue with the judge, mediation, problem-solving) and by whom (adult parties to the case, lawyers, children themselves), each of these variables affects the scope of the process, and tends towards greater or lesser complexity (in the sense defined above, as involving direct engagement with interpersonal and intra-psychic factors) in what is allowed into the social space of the courtroom. But whatever the range and depth of the 'materials' upon which processes of thinking and decision-making are based, they may still be identifiable as moral or judicial in character – or not.

The argument being advanced here chimes in with the work of certain contemporary political theorists who in different ways have tried to escape the apparent dilemma of absolutism or relativism produced by the collapse of faith in 'grand narratives' of social life. In *After Social Democracy* (1996), John Gray argues that both right-wing 'neo-liberalism' and social democracy are redundant ideologies in a globalized socio-economic environment. One consequence of this is that corporatist welfare programmes, designed to protect the population from the worst consequences of the temporary inefficiencies and inequalities generated within individual capitalist societies, are also misconceived. It is not that welfare itself has ceased to be needed, but rather that in rapidly evolving, pluralistic and complex societies, comprised of knowledgeable citizens, the ethical justifications for particular welfare practices can no longer be satisfactorily derived from the macro-political process, or legitimated only by government. Equally, in Gray's view, it cannot be left to the vagaries of markets and individual market 'choice' to determine the social fate of populations. Against this background, the urgent question is 'how can revolutionary changes in technology and the economy be reconciled with the enduring human needs for security and for forms of common life?' (Gray, 1996, p. 15). It is in the vacuum created by the impossibility of a reliance on the past, on the false certainties of tradition, or on any externally given, grand unifying socio-political framework to guide us into the future, that the 'communitarianism' espoused by Gray and others arises. A central question for communitarianism is 'From whence arises the authority for the conduct of social life?' to which Gray's answer is:

> The central insight of communitarian philosophy is that conceptions of autonomy and fairness are not embodiments of universal principles, but local understandings, grounded in particular forms

of common life....In this morality, equality is demanded as a safeguard against exclusion. It is not, in social-democratic terms, a
requirement of any theory of justice.

(Gray, 1996, p. 18)

In the political and social spheres, pluralism is accepted as a fact of
modern life, but it is not seen as a barrier to the articulation and
production of commonality or consensus. Conflicts of value are
inevitable, but the project of reconciling diversity with commonality
will require 'institution-building as well as institution-repair, along
with creativity and imagination in the making of public policy' (*ibid.*,
p. 21). Welfare policy and practice are necessarily transmuted into a
social *process*, open-ended, provisional and contested. The project of
generating ethical principles for deciding upon 'the good', from within
the ethical resources available to the culture, but in particular contexts
in which sometimes 'no common understanding exists, or in which
inherited understanding is strongly contested' is what Gray terms
'complex fairness' (*ibid.*, p. 47).

This vision derives in part from the earlier and more specific judicial preoccupations of the American philosopher Michael Walzer,
whose concept of 'complex equality' is also a response to the challenge
of pluralism or social particularity. For Walzer, as for Gray, there can
be no concept of the 'just' or the 'good' outside of the social meanings
produced within particular cultures; any universal account of these will
be practically redundant because it is divested of meanings relevant to
the specific context. Moreover, I take Walzer to be arguing that within
any society there are distinct 'spheres of justice' which are generated by
the concepts and meanings appropriate to them:

when meanings are distinct, distributions must be autonomous.
Every social good or set of goods constitutes, as it were, a distributive sphere within which only certain criteria and arrangements
are appropriate. Money is inappropriate in the sphere of ecclesias-
tical office; it is an intrusion from another sphere. And piety
should make for no advantage in the marketplace, as the marketplace has commonly been understood.

(Walzer, 1983, p. 10)

The argument of the present chapter is that the sphere of child welfare,
or even more narrowly that of child protection, can be taken as a
distinct 'sphere of justice', organized by a complex range of variables
which require an appropriately complex set of institutional, relational

and professional responses adequate to the task set by the project of 'protecting children'. I make a double use of the finding that within different but similar societies, the social arrangements for responding to child welfare and protection matters vary so widely. First, that this is in itself evidence of the kind of complexity discussed in the abstract above; but second, that once this is recognized, the creativity and diversity represented here can be a source of renewed effort in extending and deepening the capacity of any particular system, but particularly that of England and Wales, to respond to the *internal* complexity of the situations it confronts. Through an examination of some of the features of some different European systems, it is to the question of this internal complexity that I now wish to turn.

Making sense of child protection – institutional law, symbolic law and relationships

When we look at how different Western European countries think about children, families, the state and child abuse we discover that the relationship between these varies markedly, and that 'protecting children' takes on different meanings according to how these relationships are understood. Institutional, legal, and social arrangements for responding to child abuse vary accordingly. Arguably all of these institutional forms exemplify a different 'balance' between the domains of the judiciary, organized welfare and civic society, and it might be thought that this would be the basis for some kind of 'equivalence' among them; but the different social and historical configurations in each country have given rise to key institutions, which, when taken as a comparative group, appear to be *unique* to the specific national conditions which have brought them forth. This uniqueness is an outcome of social 'complexity', the product of a configuration of historical, cultural and ideological forces that mediate the functioning and development of law and welfare.

There is not space in the context of this chapter for a detailed review of the structures and modes of functioning of this variety of institutions. The reader who wants to pursue this in more depth can do so in Hetherington *et al.* (1997). However, I want to draw attention to certain specific aspects of their differences. These concern first, how and to what extent space is made within them for the 'discourse of the child'; second, the degree to which 'relationship' is a medium through which their primary aims and objectives are enacted; and third, how legal and social authority is embodied and represented within them.

These foci recapitulate the schema outlined above, of the interaction among the intra-psychic, interpersonal and social dimensions.

In France a child, as well as a parent, social worker or even a non-involved citizen can in principle request and be granted an *audience* with a Children's Judge at any time. A case of suspected child abuse can be referred to the court without legally admissible 'evidence', so long as there are clear grounds for concern. Often it is the lack of co-operation by parents with professionals already involved in worrying cases which occasions the referral. Children, including the very young, and their families, are received in the judge's office where hearings are conducted in an informal but respectful atmosphere. The judge is as much concerned with family relationships as she or he is with the detail of any abuse which has occurred; a Children's Judge can impose a range of legal orders on children, but not effect a permanent separa-tion of child from birth parents. In cases where an order is in force, a judge holds continuing individual responsibility through the duration of the order, and builds up a relationship with the child and the family. The personal dimension of children's justice is reflected in the way children talk about 'my judge' (*mon juge*), and this in turn is the title of a well-known book by a *Juge des Enfants* (Chaillou, 1989). The judge is supposed to embody, in person, the authority of the state, but also its responsibilities towards children and families; this results in the figure of the judge assuming the aspect of a benign but firm grandparent, who seeks to meld legal and symbolic authority in her or his transactions with children and their carers. Thus, the judge is bound by law, when imposing a legal order, to seek the parents' agreement to the measure he is enforcing, and a typical statutory supervision order (AEMO) will be accompanied by a package of welfare measures that it is the responsibility of the social worker to negotiate and implement. A high proportion of parents seek the continuation of such orders because they have found them helpful (Cooper *et al.*, 1995).

In France there is a highly permeable boundary between the civic and the judicial domain in matters of child welfare and protection, and juvenile crime, but what happens within the judicial sphere is not at all what happens once the same boundary is crossed in England. In the Flemish-speaking community of Belgium (Flanders) a model which is almost the inverse of the French has operated for over a decade. Here, the network of Confidential Doctor Services works on the explicit assumption that the criminalization of child abuse and the legalization of child protection works against the possibility of successfully engaging abused children, their parents (abusing and non-abusing), and the extended family or network, in working towards change in relationships and creating safe conditions for children.

Such a system relies heavily on very skilled professionals operating with clearly worked out practice methodologies and *ethically grounded norms of acceptable and unacceptable behaviour towards children*. If a guarantee of confidentiality means that abusers can approach services or risk engagement with them, this in turn means that professionals must be prepared to use their professional and moral authority to confront abusers within the context of a plan of work. Within such an approach the 'law' becomes significantly located within a domain of discretion operated by professionals, with social legitimation. It also assumes an openly pragmatic character, and is continually balanced in a fluid and evolving way with other operational criteria relevant to the total child protection task – success in engaging parents or children reduces the likelihood of eventual resort to institutional law; a strong network of extended family support offering protected living space can be deployed to reduce risks to children, in turn making it less likely that protective legal measures will be necessary; the availability of a skilled workforce, able to implement the required blend of therapeutic intervention and authority, is itself a variable which helps secure a reduced dependence on judicial measures while effectively protecting children. In this scheme of things, the severity of abuse, assessed danger and the use of law are not (as they are in England) understood according to a linear model on which 'thresholds' of risk are supposedly identifiable and accordingly trigger a range of administrative or judicial interventions. Instead, law, risk, children's capacities and wishes, family relations and the therapeutic pliability of all involved are understood as a *configuration* which must be conceived and worked with over time as a changing process (Hetherington *et al.*, 1997).

Within the confidential 'social space' created by the Flemish system of child protection, law is not denied or excluded, but relocated and reconstituted in a more organic link to social relationships. As one Flemish social worker has expressed it to me, 'We take responsibility' – for securing protection of children, confronting abusers with their responsibilities and the consequences of their actions, and restoring an adequate semblance of moral, psychological and social order in families where abuse is occurring. The Flemish system grew out of a considered assessment that institutional law was too blunt an instrument to be of much use as a central means by which to respond to the complexity of abuse and family breakdown (Marneffe, 1992). However, where the methods sketched out above reach their limits, formal institutional processes exist. First, all cases which have reached an impasse, or in which risks are judged to be too great, must be referred to a body called the Mediation Committee. This is a panel of lay people whose task is to attempt mediation in situations where children, families and professionals have become 'stuck' in their collaborative efforts. The committee has three options – to effect mediation, to refer the case to the judicial sphere or to return it to the civil sphere even though mediation has not been effective. Thus the three functions of the Mediation Committee are to act as an alternative to justice, as a filter between the civil and judicial domains, and as a buffer between the two spheres.

The committee's work is founded on the recognition that it is the state of play in *relationships* which is crucial to the matter at hand. Accordingly its own methods centre on the attempt to resolve the conflict or intransigence which is blocking progress in the effort to ameliorate children's predicaments. Beyond or 'behind' the Mediation Committee stand the courts. In so far as the social sphere occupied by the work of the Confidential Doctor Centres is a 'negotiative' space, which relies for its efficacy upon affording a considerable degree of protection for abusers *and* children from the judicial consequences of disclosure, it can function in this way only *because* it is bounded by a realm of institutional law and judicial compulsion. The use of authority by professionals in this sphere derives its potency partly from its unspoken *conditional* character; that is the background understanding of all participants that there are limits to the negotiated sphere. Institutional law functions paradoxically in this scheme of things, serving by its absence, but also through collective awareness of its potential to be activated, to bring into the realm of engagement those 'law-breakers' who would ordinarily remain in hiding from the feared consequences of disclosure and exposure. In fact this only renders transparent a situation which pertains everywhere, namely that all welfare intervention and certainly all child protection work occupies a zone of 'semi-compulsion'. Whatever its specific content or contested status, the law is always potentially in mind even when it is out of mind, ordering social relations as much by virtue of its absence in any specific context as by its presence. This is what I think the philosopher Slabov Žižek has in mind when he writes:

> The only real obedience, then, is an external one: obedience out of conviction is not real obedience because it is already 'mediated' through our subjectivity – that is, we are not really obeying the authority but simply following our judgement....
> 'External' obedience to the Law is thus not submission to external pressure, to so-called non-ideological 'brute force' but

obedience to the Command in so far as it is 'incomprehensible', not understood; in so far as it retains a 'traumatic', 'irrational' character; far from hiding its full authority, this traumatic, non-integrated character of the Law *is a positive condition of it*. This is the fundamental feature of the psychoanalytic concept of the *superego*: an injunction which is experienced as traumatic, 'senseless' – that is, which cannot be integrated into the symbolic universe of the subject....The necessary structural illusion which drives people to believe that truth can be found in laws describes precisely the mechanism of *transference*: transference is this supposition of a Truth, a Meaning behind the stupid, traumatic, inconsistent fact of the Law.

(Žižek, 1989, pp. 37–8)

Because of his Lacanian theoretical commitments, he would probably argue that law will always retain some element of the 'traumatic' as part of its character, since in this way of thinking there is always something which remains obstinately beyond symbolization and incorporation into the domain of rational social affairs. Nevertheless, returning 'Law' from the domain of the external 'incomprehensible' to the domain of social and personal responsibility and action, and thus into the domain of the therapeutic where *transference may be worked upon* rather than projected into an alienated institutional form (the Law), is what the Flemish system of child protection aims to achieve – 'We are responsible.'

In quite different ways, then, the French and Flemish child protection systems create space, not just to enable children to have better access to and be better 'heard' within judicial, and formal or informal institutional settings; but also in working to reconcile symbolic (intra-psychic) law with institutional (social) law through the medium of direct interpersonal relationships. However, I propose that even where this has proved possible, we must recognize that institutions such as the Mediation Committee, which are invested with social authority but stand outside the law, always function *in the shadow of the law*. It is a mistake of certain varieties of communitarianism to encourage the illusion that it is possible to dispense with institutional law by 'returning it to the people'. Just as Freud proposed that the individual establishes within him or herself a super-ego, a 'legal function' which originates in the child's internal identifications with the parents in which 'the shadow of the object falls upon the ego' (Freud, 1923), so we can think of a society or social institution as having a more or less comfortable and connected relationship with its own sources of authority, but not as able to dispense entirely with the 'externality' of this relationship.

Therapeutic courts and courtrooms in the mind

England and Wales differ from other European countries by separating the 'care' jurisdiction and the criminal jurisdiction, and making them the responsibility of different courts. For different but probably related reasons there is now a growing interest in the development of alternative forms of judicial process within both the juvenile justice and child protection fields. Although the Children Act 1989 went some way to modifying the most pernicious consequences of our traditional adversarial system for children, young people and families, it has proved a resistant feature of the judicial landscape. Some highly critical analyses of the children's legal system (King and Piper, 1995; King and Trowell, 1992) have been influential, but the very significant reforms of recent years have still left many unsatisfactory aspects of our system intact. The ideological and humanitarian impulses behind the movement for 'restorative justice', mediation, alternative dispute resolution, family group conferences, and so on tend to find themselves marginalized by persisting and deep-rooted structural and cultural obstacles to change. Although I would argue that more favourable conditions for the development of 'restorative justice' exist in most Western European countries than in England, a recent commentator on the European scene summarizes the position as follows:

> At present, experiments in restorative orientation must take place within a retributive or rehabilitative justice system....Mediation and community services take place within or outside the system, at varying stages in the judicial process, with a wide variety of objectives and techniques. It is a miscellaneous profusion, an odd assortment of good intentions, opportunism and clear visions.
> (Walgrave, 1996, p. 189)

This also accurately portrays the present state of affairs in English child protection work, in which family group conferences, special child protection mediation and conflict-resolution services and other 'alternatives' have evolved alongside, and knit together more or less uneasily with, the courts and the Child Protection Conference system.

Nevertheless, what all these developments share is a focus on the use of *relationship and dialogue* as the primary medium for enacting, avoiding recourse to, or providing an alternative to conventional justice. What is strikingly absent within the English child protection system, but often structurally incorporated at the heart of other European countries' systems, is an *institutional space* in which a dialogic mode of justice or conflict-resolution takes place. Both the Flemish Mediation Committee and the *audience* conducted by the French Children's Judge constitute such social 'spaces'. Typically, they occupy an intermediate position between the state and civil society, or between the domains of legal compulsion and legal voluntarism (Hetherington *et al.*, 1997). One of the interesting side effects of surveying a range of different societies' systems of justice and protection, and adopting an anthropological rather than a jurisprudential stance towards them, is that the plethora of judicial forms suddenly appears less as a 'miscellaneous profusion, an odd assortment', and much more as evidence of human and social creativity. The idea of justice as absolute or universal recedes, and its character as a differential expression of diverse unique cultural and historical processes moves to the foreground.

> The true jury of a person's peers is the people of her town. Only they, the people who have known her all her life, and not twelve strangers, can decide her guilt or innocence. And if...she has committed a crime, then it's a crime against them, not the state, so they are the ones who must decide her punishment too.
>
> (Banks, 1997, p. 151)

So says Abbott Driscoll, husband of Dolores, in Russell Banks's (1997) novel *The Sweet Hereafter*. Dolores was the driver of the school bus which crashed, killing fourteen of the town's children, and her husband is addressing Mitchell Stephens, the lawyer who attempts to persuade the bereaved parents and Dolores, to sue various town and state institutions for negligence. The plotting of this complex story turns on the actions of Nichole, a teenage survivor of the accident, also a victim (survivor) of sexual abuse by her father, who is now a party to the negligence suit. Nichole defeats both Stephens and her father through the testimony she gives about the circumstances of the accident, so that the legal case collapses. In so doing she recovers her own power to discriminate clearly between right and wrong, and between truth and lies, implicitly restoring order to the corrupted moral universe of her family and township, to which the perverse motives of those pursuing 'justice' was in her view contributing.

I have suggested above that universalist conceptions of law and justice for children and families are seriously undermined by the contemporary anthropological evidence. The evolving interaction of historical, cultural, political, legal and moral traditions in particular places gives rise to very differently configured social institutions and practices. This form of diversity and complexity is, I wish to argue, matched by actual and potential developments which generate complexity along a different axis on which are plotted the court as social institution, the family, child welfare professionals, and children themselves. This is the multi-layered world explored in Russell Banks's novel. At a more prosaic level, as Alison Diduck describes in Chapter 8, it is the changing social status of children themselves as they are increasingly (albeit ambivalently) legitimated in the public sphere which has precipitated this challenge to traditional categories of social organization and conduct. In Britain, the participation of children in the legal and welfare arena, where their own circumstances and futures are at stake, has been driven by the rights-based philosophy informing our welfare and judicial policies and practices. Where children, or for that matter adults, assume the status of rights-bearing subjects, the assumption is that they do so by virtue of a capacity for rationality, and within a rational universe of discourse wherein their rights may be exercised. But where child abuse and severe family conflict are concerned and, in particular, when the effects of abuse upon the minds of children are taken into account, then, as I shall try to show, ordinary capacities for rational thought and behaviour may be severely damaged or compromised.

If children are increasingly to enter the domain of the court as *full subjects* (which does not necessarily mean adult subjects) rather than legal objects, we may ask in turn what happens when the court enters the mind or subjectivity of the child? How (or indeed can) external 'justice' in fact 'do justice' to the experience and internal predicaments of children? What are the implications for our system of justice if in fact it transpires that the internal situation for the child is simply not capable of redress in the terms understood by conventional justice, or that the sense of justice, the capacity to think in terms of justice, has been damaged? This is the situation explored in *The Sweet Hereafter*, and represents a point of meaningful engagement between clinical psychoanalysis and the concerns of justice. I will draw on two examples as a way of exploring these questions.

In her (1994) paper 'Learning to think in a "war zone" ', Debbie Hindle describes the process of twice-weekly psychotherapy with Jamie, a nine-year-old boy who was the subject of protracted legal proceedings. At the time of referral he is living with foster parents, and the social workers believe that his mother will never agree to his adoption. After nine months Jamie's mother in fact applies to revoke the care order. After a long wait the court adjourns his case for a further six months to allow a further assessment, but a week before the hearing Jamie's mother withdraws her appeal against the care order. No hearing ever takes place. Shortly before the first hearing Hindle writes,

> I talked to Jamie about his uncertainties about what I would say in court, whether I could answer questions correctly and how I would perform under pressure. I also asked if he was concerned whether I would be able to speak on his behalf. The final question in Jamie's quiz was, 'How long does it take a house to fly to London?' I said 'What?...I don't know...it's an impossible question to answer – houses can't fly.' I then thought with him about how impossible it was for him to think about what was happening and to say where he wanted to live. At this point Jamie said, 'I don't know what to think, I don't know what I want. I don't want to have to choose...'.
>
> (Hindle, 1994, p. 348)

The laudable requirement that we should 'ascertain the wishes and feelings' of children in legal proceedings arguably also betrays an adult-centred rationalism. What if, as with Jamie, a child has absolutely *conflicting* wishes and feelings? How does the court, and judicial logic, accommodate the possibility that there is no single 'truth' to be ascertained? Debbie Hindle continues,

> Jamie was right when he said 'he didn't know what to think'. The truth of his situation seemed to be that there was more than one truth. His mother was his birth mother; his foster mother provided his 'home'. In such a situation one truth cannot eclipse the other.
>
> (Hindle, 1994, p. 352)

And later, when his mother has withdrawn her appeal,

> Jamie demonstrated how he felt the dropping of the court case was like a nasty trick....The idea that he had been cruelly tricked alternated with games in which he mimed sadistic pleasure at tricking others. Often he played out court-room scenes in which the puppets on the stand were implored to tell the *truth*, the whole truth and nothing but the truth....I said he did not know the

truth of the situation, adding, 'Jamie, between you and your mother – you might never know the whole truth of the situation.' Jamie said, 'I know.'

(Hindle, 1994, pp. 353–4)

No court system can offer guaranteed access to 'the truth', for children or adults in any judicial domain. While it is the court's responsibility in child welfare cases to reach a decision 'in the best interests of the child', there is no absolutely privileged methodology or perspective through which this can be achieved. Decisions in such cases can only be the product of a balanced and impartial assessment of a complex range of considerations, leading to (in multiple senses of the word), a judgement. While I and many others would endorse an enhanced emphasis upon the child's perspective, we must recognize that this renders the process *more complex rather than less*, and our confidence in reaching a good decision *less rather than more certain*. In essence, this is because once we expose the court and its methodologies to the realm of human feeling, suffering and general subjectivity, we also enter a realm of multiple truth, ambivalence and inherent uncertainty. In Jamie's case, as with most children in such circumstances, these conflicts and uncertainties are lodged within him, as well as between other involved parties.

In one sense this is not a new recognition. Within the adversarial English court system all contested child welfare cases take the form of institutionalized and regulated family conflicts, with representation for the various parties by lawyers and guardians *ad litem*, and the judge or bench sitting at the head of the table. Surely it is precisely the job of the courts to decide the undecidable, to take over from those with parental responsibility when they are unable to resolve their predicaments in favour of the vulnerable, the children? When Jamie says 'I don't want to have to choose', he may not only be saying 'I can't decide', but also 'Will someone please do it for me?' With the help of skilled therapy Jamie has been enabled to hold onto 'the truth' of his situation, which is that there is no single truth or predominant wish, and still recognize that a decision has to be made. This, I propose is a reasonable characterization of what it is to *have a capacity for justice*. Although he feels that his mother and the system fail him, it seems that he has an idea in his mind of what a good court would try to do – allow the truth to emerge and make a decision in impossible circumstances. However, I want to propose equally, that in many cases where the courts become involved this capacity itself has been damaged, and that this has profound implications for what the role of our institutions should be in such situations.

Justice and psychic damage

In the first part of this chapter I argued for a recognition of both the plurality and cultural specificity of judicial institutions in child welfare, but also for a much more inclusive and complex understanding of the social role of these institutions, one which extends their significance far beyond the sterile debate between 'justice and welfare'. The more unusual step I want to take at this point is to extend the metaphor of judicial process as occupying or constituting itself within a social space, by thinking about the capacity for justice, the source of creativity in the production of judicial forms, as a *space within the mind*. In *The Ego and the Id*, the paper with which Freud ushered in his late, mature, 'structural' theory of the mind, he describes the ego as a 'frontier-creature'.

> As a frontier-creature, the ego tries to mediate between the world and the id....Whenever possible, it tries to remain on good terms with the id, (but)...in its position midway between the id and reality, it only too often yields to the temptation to become sycophantic, opportunist and lying, like a politician who sees the truth but wants to keep his place in popular favour.
>
> (Freud, 1923, p.56)

This idea occurs in a famous passage in which Freud describes the ego as a 'poor creature owing service to three masters and consequently menaced by three dangers: from the external world, from the libido of the id, and from the severity of the super-ego' (p. 55). The strength or frailty of the ego derives from its greater or lesser capacity to interpose the 'processes of thinking' and submit mental processes to reality testing; and by virtue of its relation to perception, says Freud, the ego confers on mental experience an order in time. If there is a failure in the capacity of the ego to manage the conflicting demands or forces to which it is subject, the result is a rupture in the person's relation to everyday social and interpersonal realities. The function of the ego as 'frontier-creature' is to maintain an arena of *mental space* in which thinking about the relationship between inner (psychic) and outer (social and interpersonal) realities can occur.

Freud himself wrote very little about justice, and psychoanalytic models of the mind have evolved and considerably deepened since the

1920s, but the groundwork for a theory of the preconditions of justice is set out in these thoughts. Justice presupposes the capacity to think even-handedly about conflicting realities but, vulnerable to the temptation to become 'sycophantic and lying' and a poor servant of truth, is at permanent risk of corruption. This may seem a banal or obvious point, in the sense that all mature personal or social functioning depends on the capacity to negotiate dilemmas, manage conflicting feelings, attend to the emotional needs of others and so on. However, one of the contributions of a psychoanalytic understanding of social processes and institutions has been to show how often and easily these capacities are impaired, distorted or violated, particularly in the face of an emotionally painful and disturbing institutional 'task'. In the face of child abuse, arguably more than this is at stake, for much abuse both derives from and creates fundamental damage to the ability to 'think' properly about the difference between self and other, adult and child, right and wrong, or whose emotional needs and desires belong to whom. Child abuse brings us into close contact with what is popularly termed 'madness'. What is the significance of this for courts and other institutions involved with child abuse and welfare? This is my larger question at this point.

A man who had been repeatedly physically abused by his father in childhood came to a psychotherapy session one day and recounted an episode in which, at about the age of three or four, he had lost control of his bladder and bowels while on a family visit with relatives, causing his father to beat him. I linked this material with some of his behaviour in therapy and the following day he came to his session and said that he had been able to think more clearly about this memory, and now believed that events had been the other way round – his father had beaten him for some reason, perhaps because he had been pestering to go home, and he had lost control of himself as a result.

Some days later, the patient arrived and in quite a composed manner gave me an account of some events which had taken place earlier that same day. He had gone to his supervisor's office for a pre-arranged appointment, knocked on the door, and seeing that there was no-one in the room, had collapsed into a state of extreme anxiety believing that he had mistaken the day, the appointment had been yesterday and he had therefore missed it, his supervisor would now be furious and his career stood in jeopardy. He went back to his room and began writing a letter of apology, only to return to reality when the supervisor phoned up enquiring whether he was coming to the appointment. In some respects, these events recapitulated my very first meeting with the patient himself; we had arranged an appointment at a particular hour, but he arrived fifty minutes earlier, believing he was ten minutes late. Thus our first exchanges involved him apologizing to me for being late, while I had to persist gently but firmly in pointing out that he was early, until he took in his mistake.

Soon after the session described above, I thought it possible that I myself might be hard pressed to arrive at a particular session on time. Whether or not it was technically advisable in the context, I decided at the end of the preceding session to say to the patient that it was just possible I might be a few minutes late for our next appointment but that he should wait for me. When he came to this appointment (for which I arrived in good time), he was consumed with fury at me, believing that I had told him I might be late in order to manipulate the therapy, by deliberately provoking his angry feelings and in order to set him a complex test in how to react. In this state of mind there seemed to be no idea for the patient that my communication had been intended in good faith, or had anything to do with my anticipation of ordinary realities about travel and timing. I had become, temporarily, a purely malevolent and spiteful figure devoted to putting the patient on trial rather than helping him.

Much of the time and in a variety of aspects, this man's capacity for realistic everyday interpersonal and social functioning remained intact. He was able to use psychotherapeutic processes effectively, because he was able to enter into a relationship with me, in order that we could *together* work on understanding and bringing about change in the 'area' of himself which was not capable of 'realistic' functioning, but which was dominated by extreme anxiety and distorting fantasies. But in so far as he was able to co-operate with me in this task, I suggest that he was persuaded that I would give all aspects of his experience *a fair hearing*.

However, at the point at which he accuses me of 'manipulating the therapy', he is in the grip of the part of himself which is, amongst other things, convinced that I am incapable of fair and dispassionate conduct or attitude. Part of my reaction to his outburst is feeling extremely *unfairly accused* and that my motives have been systematically inverted. However naïvely from the perspective of therapeutic technique, I was trying to be helpful and protective to him. Within the therapy his outburst represents an advance; his composure is gone and instead of telling me 'about' his state of mind, he gives me a very direct experience of what it is like to be *put on trial for something I have not done, and be the object of blind, retributive judgement.*

In this state of mind, which he now succeeds in putting into me, he relies (from a therapeutic perspective) on my capacity to hang on to another kind of thinking in which I can continue to assert that there is another side to this story: however he experiences matters, I had not intended to have this effect on him. Matters are not only as he so powerfully wishes to convince me they are. To the extent that I now succeed in maintaining a stance in which 'there are two sides to this question', it is by virtue of the operation of a *third faculty, which stands apart and exercises a capacity for balanced judgement.*

Law, therapy and social reality

What are the links, if any, between the function of the therapist in a process like the above, and the actual or potential function of the courts and professionals in child welfare matters? Child abuse, particularly sexual abuse, but also severe or protracted family conflict and breakdown, serve to attack the most fundamental capacities for ordinary personal and social relationship. At worst, this represents not simply a personal and social injustice, but an assault upon and a destruction of the most basic structures of psychic and social order *upon which the possibility of justice depends.* The patient described above does, like the child Jamie, have a 'courtroom in his mind'; but unlike Jamie, in certain states there is for this man no hope of justice or truth ever emerging because the wrong people are on trial and accused. The judge cannot tell true from false, the jury is corrupt and capricious. Crucially, I think that before he begins to explore his disturbed areas in therapy, one part of him cannot properly distinguish belief from knowledge. In the grip of his punitive, self-accusatory fantasy, it is as though he *knows he is in the wrong* (or on occasions in the right), while at other times he *knows* others to be right or wrong. The capacity to believe rather than know implies the ability to entertain alternative accounts or interpretations of the same 'event', and this is what the patient achieves with respect to his experience of childhood abuse. But such states of mind, when children experience them in relation to their abuse, render the injunction to 'believe children' in their disclosures uncomfortably simplistic. It is not that we should disbelieve children either, but rather through listening to them properly, remain attentive to the deeper level at which there may be damage to the most basic capacity to either believe or disbelieve (Britton, 1995). This may come closer to doing justice to children's experience, and also validates the foundations of justice itself, which involve the ability to entertain doubt, even though this may be beyond the realms of 'reasonable doubt'.

The job of the therapist is, in one sense, to enable a recovery or restoration of a more stable psychic 'ordering', in which fantasy can be distinguished properly from reality, and a capacity for psychic truth rather than psychic confusion can be secured. Like the court, the therapist can provide no absolute guarantee of certainty in these matters, only a 'good enough' sense of psychic reality in her or himself not to be invaded and persuaded by the patient's effort to convince her or him that things are the opposite of what they actually are or can only have one possible version. Looked at another way, the therapist must have sufficient defences against her or his own propensity for psychic confusion to continue to represent what Freud termed 'the reality principle'. Courts cannot and should not try to be therapists or vice versa, but they can be more or less therapeutic in their approach to human predicaments in which the connections between intra-pyschic, interpersonal and social dimensions are central. For the abused, neglected, or traumatized child, the restoration of 'law and order' is necessarily both a private and a public issue; in therapy, as we see above, the possibility of restoring a relationship to interpersonal reality depends upon the availability of another person to 'bear witness' or act as an effective mediator between the inner world and social experience. If the law, in Žižek's terms, is not to be traumatic, incomprehensible and irrational, then it must come into direct relationship with those who have been exposed to the traumatic and irrational. In the final analysis, this is why children's participation in their own court proceedings matters. Nichole in *The Sweet Hereafter* uses the public proceedings to reassert her capacity to know the truth, to reclaim the power and psychological autonomy which her father has stolen from her. She does this by telling a lie, but the ability to tell a lie depends in its turn upon the ability to know truth from lies, which, as the novel makes clear, the abuse had compromised. 'But Daddy knew why I had lied. He knew who was normal and who wasn't. Mr Stephens couldn't ever know the truth, but Daddy always would' (Banks, 1997, p. 216).

In some spheres of justice, the responsibility of the law is to ensure that as reliable as possible an answer to the question 'true or false', 'guilty or innocent' emerges at the end of the case. In others, this is beside the point, or at least only one dimension among many equally pertinent ones. One of the most damaging aspects of England's traditions of child welfare, is the confusion of social purposes which pervades the operation of the law in these matters. Child welfare is principally concerned with questions of personal relationship, social belonging and the mental health of children, which depends upon securing the best possible resolutions of these in situations where they have been severely ruptured. The argument of this chapter thus has no simple or single conclusion, because the operation of the law as a form of social 'reality principle' must be capable, like a mature individual adult, of contending with complexity; of making decisions which are definite but also provisional, in circumstances where all the evidence is not gathered in and in which different constructions of the facts would suggest different decisions; of confronting and embracing open-ended and uncertain predicaments in pursuit of optimal but always uncertain outcomes.

11 What is good and bad sex for children?

Wendy Stainton Rogers and Rex Stainton Rogers

Recent trends in English law and practice point to a paradox. On the one hand, a fifteen-year-old boy who forces sexual intercourse upon a woman of thirty can be charged with – and indeed convicted of – rape. On the other hand, a thirty-year-old woman who actively encourages a boy of fifteen to have sex with her can be charged with and convicted of a criminal offence. In other words, an act of heterosexual intercourse between a male below the age of sixteen and a woman over the age of sixteen is treated by the law as hinging upon the behaviour of the woman concerned rather than that of the boy. The boy is seen to be capable of initiating sex with an unwilling woman – and hence, presumably, of not just merely consenting to it but of actively being culpable for his actions. But when the woman is a willing participant, then the boy is viewed as incapable of consenting – he is treated as the victim of a sexually abusive act. This strange situation highlights (and, to some extent, results from) two seemingly incommensurable concerns:

- First, that juvenile sexual offenders should not be able to escape the consequences of their actions merely by virtue of their age (and, in parallel, that their victims and society in general should not thereby be deprived of 'justice being done and seen to be done')
- Second, that juveniles are in need of special protection against being sexually exploited by a prohibition that reflects their immaturity and vulnerability to adult coercion and exploitation.

This bifurcation in approach to young people and sexuality permeates our society. Even those who advocate the legalization of sex between children and adults make a distinction between what they regard as 'consensual' and enforced sexual activity. This view was clearly expressed by Brongersma, a well-known Dutch lawyer who has written extensively in defence of this position. He argues for the need to distinguish between:

> two very different types of adult offenders [which] is essential if rational action is to follow. Broadly, these groups are, on the one hand, adults who form happy and often affectionate relationships with children and are welcomed to sexual involvement; and, on the other hand, there are adults who manipulate events undesirably by applying physical or emotional pressure.
>
> (Brongersma, 1978, p. 109)

Such apologists for paedophilia aside, few would regard small children as being able to form 'happy and often affectionate relationships' which involved sexual contact with adults. We have argued in detail elsewhere (Stainton Rogers and Stainton Rogers, 1996) that attempts to adopt such a position ignore the power differential between adults and children.

However, with what the law calls 'mature minors' (that is, young people who are still, legally, children but treated as capable of undertaking certain adult powers and responsibilities) matters are not so clear-cut. Even within the European Union there are considerable divergences (perhaps as much as six years) between the youngest and the oldest ages at which 'serious' sexual acts are either legal (in the sense that the young people involved are seen to have reached an age at which they can consent) or not pursued in the courts. Furthermore, there are a range of moderating or exacerbating conditions. For example, in some countries the age differential between the partners is taken into account; in some what is at stake is the power relationship between them. In others there are different 'ages of consent' for heterosexual and homosexual sex. It is usually, then, these older minors who feed the paradox with which we began, although not exclusively so – recently in the UK two ten-year-old boys were charged with the rape of a nine-year-old girl.

Value judgements thus become much more contentious once we begin to consider the 'grey areas' in between childhood and adulthood. Once we do, we come up against complex concerns about, for example, the competing entitlements of the young – to protection from adult exploitation and coercion on the one hand; and, on the other, to autonomy, to access to information and to be treated as authentic persons with the capacity to make choices for themselves. These, in turn, raise questions about the social construction of 'childhood', and the way the adult world may 'infantilize' the young to serve its own ends.

Arenas of adjudication

We have, thus far, loosely identified two arenas in which children and sex come under regulation: criminal law and child protection law. However, the law is not the only arena in which opinions are expressed about the rightness or wrongness of children's engagement with adults in sexual activity. Protagonists for paedophilia, as we have noted, are one such special interest group, notable for the self-serving interest of the case they make to decriminalize 'consensual' adult–child sex.

We should not assume, though, that others lack self-interest in the cases that they make. For example, among professionals and academics whose work focuses on child protection it has now become almost mandatory to assert that *any* sexual encounter between a child and an adult is, by definition, 'child sexual abuse' or, indeed, a form of incest – a term deliberately used in order to disturb. Dominelli's (1989) all-encompassing definition of incest provides a good illustration of this rhetorical strategy:

> Incest has many subtle faces. Incest can be an uncle showing pornographic pictures to a 4-year-old. It can be a father mastur-bating as he hovers outside the bathroom where his child is, or one who barges in without knocking. It can be a school bus driver forcing a student to sit with him, fondling her under her skirt at the traffic lights….It can be the way a father stares at his daughter's developing body, and the comments he makes. It can be the way an aunt caresses her nieces when she visits. It can be the forced exposure to the sights and sounds of one or both parents' sexual acts. It can occur through father and mother forcing their child to touch or be touched by other children while pictures are being taken.
>
> (Dominelli, 1989, p. 297)

A strategy like this, designed deliberately to shock the reader out of complacency, is deployed for the purpose of protecting children. But other interests are also served. In Dominelli's case her standpoint is an explicitly feminist one. In adopting such a broad definition of what constitutes incest, she is also constructing a powerful warrant for the regu-lation of adult sexuality in general (given there is one reference to women as possible abusers) and the regulation of male sexuality in particular.

By defining every instance of sexual interaction between adults and children (even those of which the child is completely unaware) as 'incest' or as 'sexual abuse', it is made self-evident that such behaviour is, by definition, 'bad sex' for children, carrying as it does connotations of exploitation and coercion. The protectionist discourse thus constructs a very clear demarcation, one where there is no leeway at all – no possibility of any form of adult–child interaction involving anything in the least sexual which could be constituted as 'good sex' for the child.

Yet by no means everybody regards, say, sex between a fifteen- and an eighteen-year-old as 'sexual abuse' and so would not see this as constituting 'bad sex' for the fifteen-year-old. Classical romances such as *Romeo and Juliet* are not seen as stories about incest, but as love stories. More crucially for today's young people, as Sullivan (1992) has pointed out, to treat a sexual relationship between an under-sixteen- and an over-eighteen-year-old as 'sexual abuse' is to pathologize a great deal of teenage behaviour (and also that of parents and others – such as doctors – who, for example, offer under-age young people access to contraception). Bremner and Hillin (1994) report that currently 48 per cent of girls and 36 per cent of boys say that they have had penetrative sex before the age of sixteen, so we are not talking here of a trivial proportion of young people.[1]

Equally, there are few who would argue that childhood masturbation is, in itself, harmful to the child concerned or intrinsically 'wrong'. Neither does the sexual play between young children arouse concern. It is seen by most people as 'harmless exploration'.

What we can see here, then, is a divide between popular wisdom and the views promoted by those who advance a strongly protectionist case. Common sense accounts distinguish between 'good' (or at least not 'bad') sex for children – which includes consensual sex between teenagers, masturbation and 'playing doctors and nurses' – and 'bad' sex – anything involving coercion, exploitation or force. The protectionist discourse, however, is much more suspicious about what may be behind the 'innocent' sexual play of small children or those teenage relationships that involve sex. Presented with these potential examples of 'good sex', protectionists are quick to point out that the children's sexual play may indicate that the children concerned have been sexualized as a result of sexual abuse, or that young men are no less capable of sexual coercion than adult men, and young women no less vulnerable to it than adult women.

The construction and energization of child sexual abuse

This protectionist discourse is of relatively recent origin. This can be observed by comparing two accounts of what we would now call 'child sexual abuse'. The first was published in the mid-1960s. In it the author, West, defined paedophilia as 'indulging in sexual play with pre-pubertal children' and says of its effects:

> Actually the dangers to children are less than popularly supposed. Most paedophiles are childish in their approaches, and go no further than the mutual display and fondling which small children might indulge in among themselves. Although this does not make the offence any less obnoxious, the fact is that the victims are not infrequently seductive, attention-seeking children who try to elicit interest from neighbours, relatives or strangers where they have not been able to get it from their own parents....Given a normal background the experience is not likely to impair a child's emotional development, although the fuss and distress of subsequent court appearances can be harmful.
>
> (West, 1967, p. 195)

Now contrast this with a description given twenty years later in what virtually became the 'bible' for people working with adult survivors of child abuse, *The Courage to Heal*:

> The long-term effects of child sexual abuse can be so pervasive that it's sometimes hard to pinpoint exactly how the abuse affected you. It permeates everything: your sense of self, your intimate relationships, your sexuality, your parenting, your work life, even your sanity. Everywhere you look you see its effects.
>
> (Bass and Davis, 1988, p. 33)

These accounts represent the prevailing standpoints of their times, and the contrast is striking. In the 1960s, the sexual molestation of children (as it tended to be called) was commonly seen as an inconsequential, relatively minor problem – if a problem at all. Most textbooks on child abuse concentrated on 'battered babies' and hardly mentioned sexual abuse at all. But by the 1980s concern about child sexual abuse had come to dominate the agenda among those professions that work with children, and to arouse almost constant attention in the media. Today it is seen as a social problem of massive proportions.

The impact of this shift has been considerable. It creates difficulties for children's emancipation. Efforts to protect children from sexual abuse and exploitation have led to policies and practice which can deny children quite fundamental human and citizenship rights. In a world in which there has been an extensive liberalization of attitudes and values, especially concerning sex (e.g. see Wilkinson and Mulgan, 1995) any countenancing of sex between adults and children has 'bucked the trend'. Children's sexuality has become a taboo topic – unthinkable and unacknowledgeable. Even those who elsewhere argue against the censorship of pornography feel they must (in public at least) draw the line at pornography involving children (e.g. see Thompson, 1994). Any attempt to argue an emancipatory case – to seek to explore the down-side costs to children and young people of protection, or to open up debate about the sexual rights of young people (such as reducing the 'age of consent' for gay young men) – can (and does) lead to accusations of, at the very least, acting (either complicitly or naïvely) as an apologist for the paedophile lobby. Yet, even at this risk, this is what we propose to do.

The discursive production of the equation child + sex = abuse

Our starting point is that child sexual abuse has been seen discursively 'knowledge into being' (cf. Curt, 1994) as a serious social problem within a history of broader regulatory strategies over childhood sexuality. As we have described elsewhere (Stainton Rogers and Stainton Rogers, 1992), in the nineteenth century the 'big issue' was masturbation (or self-abuse, as it was commonly called). Child experts of the time used powerful rhetorical strategies to justify their calls for its control. Not only, they argued, was masturbation 'bad' in a moral sense of being wrong. It was also 'bad *for*' children – harmful and damaging to them. This is well illustrated in medical texts of the period, such as Walling's *Sexology* (1909). Walling asserted that child masturbators stood out as different from other children. Detecting the self-abused child, he claimed, was something anyone could do by following a simple checklist of symptoms: 'Prominent characteristics are, loss of memory and intelligence, morose and unequal disposition, aversion or indifference to legitimate pleasures and sports, mental abstractions, stupid stolidity, etc.' (Walling, 1909, p. 38). Where these signs were manifested, Walling argued, they provided evidence that masturbation has done its evil work. Quoting with approval a contemporary medical authority, he noted:

> Deslandes says: 'I have every reason, from a great number of facts presented to me in practice, that of every twenty cases of leuchorrhea (whites), or of inflammation of the vulva or vagina in children [sic] and young girls, there are at least fifteen or eighteen which result from masturbation!'.
>
> (Walling, 1909, p. 46)

But the harm resulting from self-abuse was, he said, not just a short-term matter. Self-abuse laid 'the foundation of physical, mental and moral maladies' (*ibid.*, p. 34) in adult life. Thus the medical discourse of the time provided a potent justification for regulation. The self-abusing child needed to be identified, so that the short- and long-term harmful effects of masturbation could be tackled. Anti-masturbatory devices were used, and where these failed it was not unusual to resort to surgery.

However, the spotlight of concern gradually got shifted away from masturbation. By the 1940s and 1950s its perceived harmfulness was much diminished. It came to be seen as a natural stage in development, out of which a child will grow so long as parents do not take it too seriously. By the 1960s it came to be seen as 'natural' and 'healthy'. For instance, the baby-care guru of the time, Benjamin Spock, offered this advice to parents:

> It's better not to give him [sic] the idea that he is bad or his genitals are bad. You want him to go on having a wholesome, natural feeling about his entire body....At three it's related to his feelings....We realize now that there is a childish kind of sexual feeling at this period, which is an essential part of normal development.
>
> (Spock, 1963, p. 368)

The same kind of liberatory treatment of children's sexuality was shown in texts specifically directed to 'sex education', and continued to be viewed as acceptable up until the early 1980s, as this idealized child–parent interaction for five- and six-year-olds by Calderone and Ramey shows:

Why does my body feel funny and my bottom jerk after I've rubbed my clitoris (penis) for a while?

Because when you play with it long enough to feel really good the muscles around your genitals get excited. Then something pleasurable happens we call an orgasm, or a climax...

Jimmie and I were playing doctor. He said I should kiss his sore penis to make it well. Would it be okay to do that?

Kissing is one of the ways we pleasure each other, when we know and trust each other very well.

(Calderone and Ramey, 1982, p. 64)

For sex educators during that period, when 'responsible emancipation' was seen as the ideal solution to the equation child + sex = ?, 'good sex' for children was seen to meet the following 'mission statement':

Throughout childhood boys and girls learn to know and experience their own bodies, each with its own unique sexual repertoire. This is the only way they can grow to understand, in later years, that sex can be a component in a mutually respectful, loving relationship. The ability to share sexual intimacy with another person and to make intelligent use of our reproductive potential requires that you behave responsibly toward your partner as well as yourself. Full and open opportunity throughout childhood is essential for such awareness and such a capacity to be developed.

(Calderone and Ramey, 1982, p. 4)

Today such text is highly discomforting to read. As Gerrard (1997) has pointed out, writing about 'kiddie' beauty competitions, 'our sense of childhood has become sexualized; we are perturbed by images that once we found simple'. It is no longer possible to read text such as the above or look at images of childhood innocence without some disquiet.

None of the Miss Pears from 1958 onwards has ever been sexy: their images guard the sanctity and chastity of youth. Like the golden boy in the Millais 'Bubbles' painting, they are lispy, thumb-sucking, winsome, adorable, nostalgic and wholesome images of a picture-book childhood. A far cry from Freud, you might think. And yet, of course, we are all post-Freudians now. The children are innocent, but we are not. We know all about

John Berger's ways of seeing – we have an ambiguous and corrupted gaze. We know too much about child abuse, paedophiles, prurience and perverted adult desire to be entirely comfortable with the cute Miss Pears.

(Gerrard, 1997, p. 5)

In other words, we are no longer prepared to countenance the possibility that there may be any kind of sex that is 'good' for children.

Even in the earlier, more 'innocent' 1960s, regulation of childhood sexuality did not cease. But what is notable about the situation pre-1980 is that this regulation was directed towards the sexuality of the young themselves – the teenage girl who became pregnant was seen as a 'social problem', likely to be institutionalized in a mother and baby home, and expected to give the child up for adoption or put under pressure to marry. Regulation was achieved, then, by drawing a very clear distinction between childhood and adulthood, and constituting 'real' sex (i.e. sex-for-real rather than 'innocent and childish' exploration) as prohibited and proscribed to children. Adult–child sexual activity was subject to strong prohibition, but since it was generally regarded as a rare aberration, it was not seen to merit significant institutional regulatory effort.

By the 1980s, however, mainly as a result of second-wave feminism coupled with a broader movement to counter 'child abuse' (arising from a growing recognition of children's rights and a lessening of parental authority, together with increased state surveillance of and intervention in families), the 'sexual abuse' of children came to be seen as far more widespread and common. Since the early 1980s there has been a dramatic increase in the number and proportion of cases of child sexual abuse reported and investigated. Parton *et al.* (1997) report that whereas in 1978 only eighty-nine children were listed in England on child protection registers because of concerns about sexual abuse, by 1986 this figure rose to nearly 6,000 and by 1994 it reached 9,600.

It was in 1987 that child sexual abuse first became headline news in the UK, when a total of 197 children were removed from their parents in Cleveland, largely as a result of medical examinations by two paediatricians and an interventionist strategy developed by the local authority. More recently still, attention has refocused again. While the UK government advocates a 'lighter touch', with fewer investigations and more family support work (Rose, 1994), the 'horror stories' now making headlines are child pornography and child prostitution.

As Gerrard (1997) points out, we live in a time when it is no longer possible to see sex (alongside other adult 'vices') as 'off limits' for children, for nowadays:

> [c]hildren have sex, have children (in the last few weeks there seems to have been a spate of 12-year-old mothers), take drugs, commit crimes – behave, that is, like adults themselves, as if all the boundaries have been erased.
>
> (Gerrard, 1997, p. 5)

Increasingly this censorship of childhood sexuality takes the form of simply denying it, and refusing to accept that there can be any form of sex that is 'good' for children on account of the terrible harm that is wrought by any kind of sexual experience in childhood.

What is going on?

Strong parallels can be drawn between the medical discourse of the early part of this century and that of today. Both assert the short- and long-term harmfulness of children's involvement in sexual activity, and use this harm-warrant to justify intervention to prevent or stop it. However, where the discourses differ is in their location of 'the problem'. For instance, while Walling (1909) acknowledged that masturbation was often the result of 'instruction' (generally he saw the culprits as older children or female carers such as governesses or nursemaids) he sited the cause of harm within *the child's* masturbatory activity itself. The acts of others were accorded very little interest – mere sidelines to his main preoccupation with the child's own actions as the site of vice. In contrast, today masturbation is viewed as, at most, no more than a symptom of the *real* cause of the harm – the sexual abuse to which the child has been subjected.

Similar events and phenomena are thus clearly being construed in quite different ways. In the early twentieth century it was *self*-abuse which was *the* problem and any involvement by another person merely a side-issue of little consequence. In the 1980s and 1990s it is abuse *of the child* which is *the* problem, and any masturbation in which the child engages nothing more than one of any number of signs that may alert the well-informed carer or practitioner that the child may be at risk.

So, we can ask, what is going on? Why is it that while the locus of concern gets shifted, the product of child + sex arouses so much hostility? Some clues are provided by Foucault (1990, original French 1976), who argued against the popular view that the twentieth century has brought forth a liberalization of sexuality. He suggested that what has happened was not so much deregulation as the replacement of one set of regulatory strategies by another. Sexuality was one of the main targets for Foucault's critical analysis within his three volumes of a *History of Sexuality*. In Volume I he asserted that:

> Sexuality must not be thought of as a kind of natural given, which power tries to hold in check, or as an obscure domain which knowledge tries gradually to uncover. It is the name given to a historical construct; not a furtive reality that is difficult to grasp, but a great surface network in which the stimulation of bodies, the intensification of pleasures, the incitement to discourse, the formation of special knowledges, the strengthening of controls and resistances, are linked to one another, in accordance with a few major strategies of knowledge and power.
>
> (Foucault, 1990, pp. 105–6)

Under modernism, he argued, sexuality operates in a highly potent relationship with power, via a 'regime of power-knowledge-pleasure'. Foucault saw sexuality as an 'especially dense transfer point for relations of power' (*ibid.*, pp. 104–5) and, given the potent instrumentality with which sex is imbued, he suggested that a number of strategies have been developed for its regulation. These include: the hystericization of women's bodies; the socialization of procreative behaviour; the psychiatrization of perverse pleasure; and the pedagogization of children's sex. Such strategies, he contested, are used to control sexuality and 'mask its more indiscreet, conspicuous and intractable aspects'. But they are also the means by which sexuality is itself *produced*. What we see and portray, debate and agonize over as 'sexuality' is the product of the strategies we use to address its potential for the wielding of power, and its counter-pole, resistance.

Here we will concentrate upon exploring the strategy of 'pedagogizing' the sexuality of childhood. This strategy can be seen both as problematizing and seeking to regulate children's sexuality. These can be viewed as responses to the potential of childhood sexuality to act as a site of resistance to adult power. Foucault writes of the 'precious and perilous, dangerous and endangered potential' (1990, p. 104) of childhood sexuality, which, being both 'natural' and, at the same time, 'contrary to nature', 'poses physical and moral, individual and collective dangers'. Consequently, he argues: '[t]he sex of children has become, since the eighteenth century, an important area of contention around which innumerable institutional devices and discursive strategies have been deployed' (*ibid.*, p. 30).

Foucault asserted that we can see this manifested, for instance, in the architecture of schools, designed to expose children to constant and vigilant scrutiny. More generally, the strategy places all those in authority over children in a state of perpetual alert, and exhorts them to control the sexuality of the children in their care. In Foucault's (1990) analysis, what this demonstrates is the way in which our society has – he argues, for the first time in history – assembled a machinery for 'speechifying, analysing and investigating' children's sexual activity.

Arguments for liberalization

Foucault can hardly be seen as a 'neutral observer' in all this (as others, such as Bell, 1993, have examined in detail). In 1978, together with Guy Hocquenghem and Jean Denet, he took part in a debate arguing for the decriminalization of adult–child sexual activity (their arguments are contained in a collection of Foucault's interviews edited by Kritzman, 1988). It was a contestation against, in particular, the way that the law in France was coming to be used to constitute and police a boundary between adults and children in terms of sexuality. Their concern, in particular, was to challenge the way in which adult interest in children as sexual objects had been rendered a 'monstrous' crime and the adults so disposed had been rendered 'monsters':

> The overall tendency of today is indisputably not only to fabricate a type of crime that is quite simply the erotic or sensual relationship between a child and an adult, but also, since this may be isolated in the form of a crime, to create a certain category of the population defined by the fact that it tends to indulge in those pleasures. There then exists a particular category of pervert...of monsters whose aim in life is to practice sex with children.
> (Hocquenghem, in Kritzman, 1988, p. 277)

Hocquenghem made clear that they were only arguing against 'indecent acts not involving violence' and 'incitement of a minor to commit an indecent act' (specific definitions of offences under French law at the time). 'We were extremely careful not to touch on the question of rape, which is totally different' (*ibid.*, p. 283). Thus for this position, consent is crucial.

Consent, sexuality and power

What we can identify as going on, then, is contestation around the pivot of *consent*. This debate is of relatively recent origin, given that developmental theorization about children's sexuality has, until recently, dominated both popular and professional understandings. In the nineteenth century child experts viewed any form of child sex or sexuality, including any kind of sex play, as morally wrong, so consent was not an issue. But, as we have noted earlier, by the early twentieth century there was a liberalization of views, notably through psychoanalysis and anthropological and zoological theorization. In pointing to the 'naturalness' of childhood sexuality and to its role in the 'healthy' development of the child, consent was not an issue here either, since the naïveté of this theorization assumed that the very 'naturalness' of the sex rendered it benign.

As psychology (and sexology) strove for scientific respectability, childhood and adolescent sexuality became a matter of quantification, used to construct models of bio-social development. Early theorization about the bio-social development of sexuality was challenged because its behavioural focus, its concern for physiological grounding, and its use of animal models took no account of human subjectivity. This criticism led to the cognitive revolution of the late 1950s. It was this which brought up the issue of consent, with developmental theorists seeking to construct models of how children, as they mature, gain the capacity to reason and make moral judgements.

The debate over consent then opened up, as this theorization was subjected to criticism that it is patriarchal, heterosexist and opaque to issues of power. In portraying the capacity to consent or refuse sexual advances as an individual, developmentally acquired capability, the cognitive developmental model treats consent as nothing more than the performance of intellect – a performance that can be operated outwith gender, age and race relations.

Such critiques, initially arising from feminist commentators such as Nelson (1987) sought to counter arguments that children are 'seductive' or 'knowing' – that is, capable of not just consent but also of initiating and inviting sex with adults (as demonstrated, for example, in the description by West, quoted earlier). The advocacy of the case that children are, by definition, incapable of consent is not based upon a developmental understanding of their intellectual capabilities, but on a sensibility to their vulnerability to adult power. Their inability to give informed consent then came to be used as the basis for one of the most commonly used definitions of what constitutes child sexual abuse:

> The involvement of dependent, developmentally immature children and adolescents in sexually abusive activities they do not fully comprehend, and to which they are *unable to give informed consent*, or that violate the social taboos of family roles.
>
> (Schecter and Roberge, 1976, p. 60, emphasis added)

The assumption that children are incapable of consenting to sex with adults (or just as importantly with other children) is, however, highly problematic. In other domains, children are being seen, as they mature, as increasingly capable of participating in decision-making about matters which affect them. Indeed, this has been ratified as a right both by the United Nations Convention on the Rights of the Child, and the England and Wales Children Act 1989. Under present law in the UK, Canada and the USA, children have recently been given greater freedom to give informed consent for themselves (e.g. to being prescribed contraception) and to refuse consent (e.g. to a court-ordered medical examination), though there are notable exceptions.

However, Sullivan (1992) advises caution over reading into these recent changes in the law a commitment to promoting the emancipation of children. Rather, he suggests, what we are seeing is a medicalizing of adolescent sexuality, whereby control is shifted not from parents to children, but from parents to doctors. In other words, there is no let-up to the regulation of children's sexuality, merely a shift of regulatory power from one location to another. Despite the rhetoric of 'children's rights', Sullivan argues that, in fact, the current climate of opinion is one where this discourse is effectively silenced with regard to children's sexual rights. Writing about the consultation process which led to new legislation in Canada (Bill C-15), he noted:

> the single biggest failure of the whole reform effort was the failure to come to grips with how young people engage in sexual relations with each other, and how adults and families deal with the sexuality of young persons.
>
> (Sullivan, 1992, p. 152)

This is a response to his observation that, while there were claims at the start of the consultation procedure for the drafting of this new legislation that the committee would examine the full diversity of competing viewpoints, in fact what happened is that the 'protectionist' lobby effectively dominated the debate. The only proponents for children's rights heard by the committee were young people recruited by paedophile organizations. Not surprisingly, this allowed their arguments to be dismissed. Sullivan commented:

> The attempt to render mute...any question of a young person's sexual expression by casting it into the shady corners of paedophilia is hardly the balanced treatment of the developing legal position of the young person as an actor promised by the committee.
>
> (Sullivan, 1992, p. 82)

This is not an isolated example. Sullivan points out that something similar happened in the debates about lowering the age of consent in Australia, where once again the two competing discourses were not treated equally either in the formal process of consultation or by the press. The protectionist discourse tended to be expressed in terms of the vulnerability of small *children*; while the liberatory discourse was deployed in terms of the activities and agency of *young people*. In this way the potential problems over limiting the autonomy of young adults were neatly side-stepped. The liberatory arguments were countered by focusing on deviant sexuality – such as prostitution and paedophile exploitation. The issue of young person's sexuality – qua sexuality – was simply not allowed to be raised.

So we have a situation, certainly throughout the English-speaking world, where the protectionist discourse has come to dominate the way virtually all 'right-thinking' people view any engagement by children in sexual activity. It is also at the core of the policies and practice of welfare work with children. This protectionism is largely based on two main harm-warrants:[2]

- Concern about the psychological and emotional harm that children suffer as a consequence of sexual abuse
- Fear of the predation by paedophiles, which is seen to pose serious risks to children.

We would suggest, however, that these harm-warrants are not only much less justified than they are generally held to be (see O'Dell, 1997), they also obscure concerns which are much less altruistic – concerns about the potential for wielding the power inherent within sexuality. If we look to the power-potential of children's sexuality, then, we believe, we get a rather different story of what is going on.

It needs to be acknowledged that the case as put by the paedophile lobby is highly disingenuous over the issue of power. This is clearly highlighted, for example, by comparing the discourse of the 'Mills & Boon' genre of romantic tales with similar publications produced for the paedophile market. In the latter the clichés that trip off the page are couched in a discourse of powerful domination over a willing and acquiescent Other. This is visible in the use of phrases such as 'his shy *surrender* to my caresses'; '*yielding* to my passion'; 'he fell back in playful *submission*' – coupled with images of boys possessing an adult sexual knowingness and receptivity to seduction (albeit one which must be won over), and an imminent sexuality which is aroused by the seducer.

What this brings out is the extent to which consent in respect to sex does not operate in the same kind of a sanitized domain as, say, consent to medical treatment. Engaging in sex is seldom a matter of cool evaluation of the possible implications – a cerebral cost-benefit analysis of the options to give or withhold consent. It is, even where no overt coercion is involved, often connected with persuasion, entice-ment and 'leading on'. Indeed, sex which does not involve 'seduction' is, for many, 'bad sex' by definition – cold, unfeeling, and lacking in romance. This judgement is, of course, also laid upon adult sex outside of a romantic or relational warrant.

It is this very capacity of sex to entice and seduce which we believe is much more salient to adult sensibilities around children and sex than most would allow. For all the moralizing of protectionism within the discourse of child welfare, elsewhere children are frequently portrayed as sexualized objects, and then used to sell everything from insect repellent to designer jeans. The furore over, say, the Calvin Klein advertising campaign (in which pubescent girls and boys were shown in 'seductive' poses with their underwear showing) illustrates how blatant this has become. In the eyes of (predominantly male) adver-tisers, the juxtaposed tension of children's innocence/knowingness encapsulates a look of the 'naughty but nice', the 'look-but-don't-touch', the 'sweet but deadly' which sells, and sells very effectively.

This is not just a matter of the overt portrayal of the 'saucy school-girl' as 'jail-bait' in pornography (and its lesser vehicles, such as *Sun* and the *Sunday Sport*). Similar (though somewhat more subtly staged) images are to be found in fashion magazines, on record sleeves and birthday cards. Markers of female childhood – gym slips, a wide-eyed 'innocent' gaze, thumb-sucking, a gangly pubescent stance – have become recognizable markers of latent and inviting, yet forbidden (and therefore all the more seductive) sexual allure. Current 'cat-walk' models and their tutors are well versed in the use of such 'body language' to marshal attention through 'visceral clutch'.[3]

In other words, the adult world is well aware of the capacity for children to be – or at least be seen as (and, perhaps, to know they are seen as) – sexual. And it is, in certain settings, only too ready to exploit that sexuality. However, what it does not want to allow is for children to act as agents of their own sexuality, for this poses a number of threats. As with the sexuality of women and 'black' peoples, the dominant symbolic order needs to regulate the sexuality of children to prevent it from 'getting out of hand' (that is, posing any challenge or acting as a means of resistance).

This is where, we believe, one gets into the broader issue of how childhood itself is constituted in our time and place. Childhood is not a singularity existing in splendid isolation. Rather, it draws its meaning from contrasts with and differences from other conditions. It is the borderline of childhood/adulthood which most concerns us here and it is at that boundary that regulation becomes both most acute and most problematic. Sullivan (1992) points out that the protectionist discourse is used not only to justify taking action against the exploitation of small children, but also to justify controlling the sexuality of teenagers. Sullivan gives the example of how Canadian law now criminalizes sex between, say, a sixteen-year-old young woman and an eighteen-year-old young man, if the young man is in a position of authority over her. Law and policy in the English-speaking world seem increasingly tempted into such extensions of regulation wherever issues of power are detected.[4] The cost to young adults and adolescents is, for example, to deny them access to information (such as sex education) and confidential advice. In particular, it exposes large numbers of teenagers to forms of intervention which deny their civil rights, drawing them into a 'child protection' system which allows them little or no say in what happens to them.

Conclusion

In almost any other setting those of us who seek to challenge the hegemony of welfare professionals and the authoritarianism of their intervention can gain support from critical academics. We are concerned that in the context of sexuality and the young such a challenge is very difficult to mount. Even to raise the possibility that there may, just, be some forms of sex which are 'good' for children and that not all sexual experiences prior to the 'age of consent' are necessarily 'bad' is to call down the disapprobation of the vast majority not only of professionals working in the field of child welfare, but also of those academics active in this field.

Part of the reason is undoubtedly the 'ambiguous and corrupted gaze' arising from our exposure to feminist polemic on the misuse of male power, and to the catalogue of horrors opened up to us by the first-hand accounts of incest survivors. We can no longer make jokes about scoutmasters and vicars, pretending that all that is at stake is the gropings of a few inadequate and pathetic individuals. We know now about the regimes of coercion that allowed, for example, hundreds if not thousands of children and teenagers to be systematically raped in residential care, often over periods of several years. We know too where such abuse can lead – to bodies buried, still bound by the instruments of torture, in a garden in Gloucestershire and to little girls who starved to death in a cellar in Belgium.

But, we believe, we have to resist being beguiled into the 'knee-jerk' reactions such horrors generate. Not only do we need to recognize that there are serious down-side costs to adopting any totalizing discourse on children and sex, but we also need to acknowledge that our reactions are, themselves, not simply humanitarian. How far, we need to ask, are adults solely concerned with the 'welfare of the child'? Could it be, for example, that we are also scared and threatened by the possibilities of what might happen if children get to challenge adult authority seriously? Are we, perhaps, even jealous of such possibilities? Once again, Gerrard sums up this anxiety very neatly:

> Now, children have become dangerous to us. We are scared of their sexual precocity and their violent instincts, and we have made them into society's scapegoats....We sentimentalize them...and abhor them...and are hopelessly confused about them. We want to protect them and want to be protected from them. We think they are sweet and we think they are terrifying. We love them while...they are charmingly playing at being adults, but when they take a few steps towards adulthood, we get scared and angry and morally censorious.
>
> (Gerrard, 1997, p. 5)

To acknowledge that children may be sexual, may enjoy sex, may *use* sex as adults do is scary. But the fear will not simply go away if we pretend these possibilities do not exist. In a world in which we expose children to sexual imagery and use their images to convey sexuality, we have to find ways of confronting these possibilities, however uncomfortable that may be. This chapter is intended as a cautious beginning to that process.

Notes

1 Validating such data is notoriously problematic. The point here is that the figures point to a non-trivial proportion whether the errors lead to under- or over-estimation.

2 The concept of a harm-warrant refers to the use of purported evidence of contingent and subjective harm to warrant the regulation of activities that may not be physically damaging.

3 Visceral clutch is a useful term employed by sexologists to refer to the disturbing bodily pleasures evoked by erotica.

4 Power is, of course, an important analytic in much recent social theorizing but it is also a weasel word as easily employed for ideological purposes as 'witchcraft' or 'bourgeois'.

12 Identity, religious fundamentalism and children's welfare[1]

Stephen Frosh

Inside and out

I am writing here as a liberal humanist academic who is also a member of the traditional orthodox Jewish community in Britain. I realize that this might seem like a contradiction in terms. Liberal academics espouse critical, rational modes of thought; orthodox religious groups displace these with revelation and authority-based directives. Liberal humanism is based on a democratic urge, however well or badly one thinks that might have been achieved. Religious orthodoxy is not democratic: one cannot vote on religious practices, one can only obey the teachings as these have been passed down through religious authorities, who lay claim to their authority on various bases (charisma, learning), but mostly on the basis of *who* (what previous authority) has conferred it upon them. Yet, I doubt that this contradiction is a real, or at least a complete, one and I think the common failure to imagine the way these apparently contradictory positions come to be held together is one of the contributory factors to supporting genuine authoritarianism in religion – what is usually called fundamentalism. I think that part of what we do as liberals, humanists, secularists, and so on is to construct religious membership in such a way that it tends towards fundamentalism. Yet what actually exists in many religious communities – what differentiates them from fundamentalist, authoritarian structures – is a healthy *uncertainty* about truth. Despite rabbinical statements, a poll of the members of my own orthodox synagogue would reveal enormously varied views on everything to do with religion, from the position of women to the existence of God. Membership of a minority religious community is not the same thing as adherence to all the views and values propagated by the religious leaders of that community, however strongly stated those might be.

From the outside, however, which is the way most people look both at so-called 'fundamentalism' and at 'other' cultures, it is difficult to see how divergent and discrepant the inside might be – how multifarious a community which *appears* homogeneous might be. From the outside, appreciation of the diversity of belief and opinion which actually characterizes cultural and religious communities is often swamped by a search for simple defining characteristics; this search has strong racist undertones and it also effectively subjugates minority voices within these exoticized communities. This is one reason why real fundamentalism is so hard to engage with and contest: criticisms of fundamentalist authorities rarely build on the debates that actually take place within religious communities, but rather tend to collapse all members of those communities into one category. The result is an impoverished response to the challenge presented by fundamentalism's powerful appeal: just as fundamentalism tends to rely on simple true/false, them/us polarities, so do its opponents. As Gita Sahgal and Nira Yuval-Davis (1992) note in their introduction to the book *Refusing Holy Orders*, black women's opposition to the attacks on Salman Rushdie after the publication of *The Satanic Verses* was not just sidelined, it was also constructed as illegitimate by the discourse of multiculturalism, because it seemed to be attacking the right of Muslims to defend their religious heritage. Paradoxes of this kind, in which liberal secularists have recognized religious orthodoxy as the defining characteristic of 'other' cultures, and hence have played a part in obscuring dissenting voices within ethnic and religious communities, have led to disenchantment with multiculturalism amongst many in the anti-fundamentalist movement.[2] It is not just that multiculturalism now looks anaemic in the face of the extreme certainties peddled by evangelical fundamentalists, it also looks morally and philosophically inept, accepting as legitimate the most intolerant of religious outlooks in the mistaken (perhaps racist) belief that they represent the 'authentic' voice of 'other' cultures.

The fundamentalist order

Recently, the popular imagination has ceased to regard fundamentalism as quaint. In the light of 'Islamic terrorism', of the Rushdie affair, of the evangelical poison of the American Christian 'New Right', and of the murderous actions of members of right-wing Jewish sects, the frightening reality of militant fundamentalism has become apparent. I use the word 'reality' here without constructivist irony or relativism. I think this is the correct reading of the militant fundamentalist story; that is, it is the truth about this 'truth'. Fundamentalism of this kind is frightening, for those of us with some affiliation to specific cultural and religious groupings as well as to the purely secular world. It is frightening because of its certainty and its refusal to tolerate difference or opposition; it is frightening because it allows no space between agnosticism and its own particular brand of religion, and because it is also willing, at the extremes, to snuff out dissent if it can.

Fundamentalism is also frightening because it is seductive, offering a haven of sorts to those who are struggling to deal with what post-modernists have accurately described as the increasing fragmentation of contemporary social life. In this regard, fundamentalism can be seen to draw on the same anti-modern tendencies that fuel fascism and nationalism, movements with which it has many affinities. It is possible, indeed, that all these movements are thrown up in their modern form precisely by the sense of turmoil and disconnection which can be seen as the subject matter of postmodernism itself. Postmodernism has effectively debunked the modernist assertion that truth can be uncovered solely through the operations of reason, instead demonstrating the constant presence of forces outside of whatever can be articulated and fully known (e.g. see Žižek, 1991; also Frosh, 1997). Fundamentalism can be seen as one response to this crisis of rationality, to the despair of modernity, emphasizing revelation, authority and utopianism as a way of channelling emotion and guiding people into a state in which they feel there is sufficient certainty and order in the world. Fundamentalism thus offers a refuge from the frag-mentation produced by the conditions of late capitalism, a fragmentation of which it is itself a symptom. Moreover, when nothing can be fully understood or properly known and controlled, fundamen-talist prophecy, with its notion of a 'return in the future' through messianic redemption, becomes a rock to hold onto, a hard and stable place when everything else slips away.

If fundamentalism is fuelled by the fragmenting processes produced under the conditions of late modernity, it also shares many concerns with feminism, even though the values of the two movements are in most respects diametrically opposed. Indeed, particularly in the context of Christian fundamentalism, it has often been noted that the focus of fundamentalism is on ground marked out as important by feminists. Sexuality, fertility, women's private space, the importance of every personal act and encounter – these are shared issues. 'The personal is political' might be a fundamentalist as well as a feminist slogan, for fundamentalist injunctions touch every last corner of behaviour and thought. Every individual act is a social act, every aspect of private life is regulated, every belief prescribed.

Of course, fundamentalism is in actuality no more feminist than it is postmodernist. My point, however, is that it represents a response to some of the same issues to which postmodernism and feminism are also responding – albeit with very different political and moral trajectories. These issues include the difficulty of believing in a rational world-view as a 'grand narrative' of existence; the fragmentation of social life producing uncertainty over roots; the awareness of 'multiple identities' and the concomitant difficulty of forging an integrated sense of self; the apparent randomness of world events, despite their capacity to touch – and destroy – the lives of 'ordinary people'; the ambiguities of power and the sense that it does not inhere anywhere, yet has immense effects; and the sense of tragedy, degradation and annihilation being just around the corner. Added to these is an intense anxiety over what will become of one's own children, what path they might forge through the ravaging distractions of the contemporary world. Modernism's response to this situation is to acknowledge the pervasiveness of ambiguity – to theorize and struggle with uncertainty, contradiction, fragmentation, in the hope of finding something meaningful inside it. Postmodernism and contemporary feminism, on the other hand, both use the contradictory elements in modernity to argue for a deconstruction of the modernist belief in rationality, revealing its power structures and displaying these through theoretical and practical critique. Whilst this is an important and indeed necessary process, one result of it is more fragmentation and uncertainty, another turn of modernity's screw. Fundamentalism responds to these forces, to this great challenge, in a time-honoured way: it announces that it possesses the solution to all contemporary problems – indeed, to all *conceivable* problems – in the form of divinely revealed truth.

Describing fundamentalism

In this light, how might we begin to describe fundamentalism and the issues it raises for 'moral agendas' in relation to children? Rather than attempt a full definition, so risking replication of the assumption of homogeneity with which I started, it is easier to think of some of the elements which constitute a fundamentalist movement. First, and most importantly, there is acceptance of the existence of absolute authority. I focus on 'authority' rather than truth, because it is a distinctive characteristic of fundamentalism that its access to truth is through authority, and not through the dictates of personal conscience or the activities of the individual mind. For example, one of the debates in the orthodox Jewish community is concerned with the difference between an ethical position which states that Judaism is really about looking after people, showing moral concern, being a 'light to the nations' in the way in which personal relations are conducted; and an authority-based position which states that Judaism is not about that at all. It is about following certain laws, laws which are immutable, literally God-given. Faced with the choice between authority and insight, the fundamentalist chooses authority every time. In fact, there is an enormous religious literature about mystery, concerned with the necessary limitations of human understanding when faced with the grandeur of God – about not understanding the reasons for certain events and laws, but nevertheless accepting and obeying them. Using the Jewish example again, one of the constant appeals in the orthodox community is to a phrase found in the Bible with reference to the Children of Israel's acceptance of God's Law: *Na'aseh Ve-Nishmah*, 'We will do and we will hear' – the doing first. We agree to do it, to abide by the Law, even before we hear what it is; certainly before we think about it.

This is the determining feature of the second and perhaps more familiar attribute of fundamentalism: adherence to a sacred text or texts. Often, this is thought of as a literalist adherence, but this is an error: all sacred texts require interpretation, and it is the authority of the interpretation which fixes it in place as the legitimate way to read the text. Members of fundamentalist Jewish sects rely on rabbinic interpretations of the written text, constantly reapplied to the demands of contemporary life by the leaders of these sects. Similarly, the application of particular (selected) biblical and Koranic injunctions under contemporary conditions – surrounding homosexuality or abortion, for example – require authoritative interpretation of the texts, not just literal reading. 'Ownership' of the holy texts therefore becomes crucial in terms of the political consequences of the texts themselves.

Fundamentalism is commonly, perhaps increasingly but certainly not universally, militant; often this is evangelical militancy, but it is usually most focused within its own religion. Possessing the absolute truth and the authority to interpret it, fundamentalists of this kind cannot tolerate the existence of alternative views, other ways of portraying the teachings. Moreover, most fundamentalist sects believe that it is their task to represent the word and to root out evil alternatives, in defence of the honour and integrity of the deity. Other views are attacks, to be destroyed; authority is always maintained. Even non-militant forms of fundamentalism, such as most Hasidic groups, have numerous subtle or explicit ways of excluding dissenting voices from the community – for instance, through social and rabbinic pressure, and shunning the people involved. Interestingly, fundamentalist sects seem not to be anti-modern in every sense; they are particularly adept at using technology (witness the Iranian Mullahs, the Christian evangelists in the USA, and the Lubavitch movement), and where they can – in Iran, in Israel, in the USA – employing the power of the state. Above all, despite the responsibility placed on each individual to uphold the creed, they are collective rather than individualistic movements; they are specifically anti-humanist. In a move guaranteed to appal the liberal imagination, fundamentalists deny that the individual human subject is the highest value; preservation of the truth is more important. Hence the culture of martyrdom and violence to be found in many of the more extreme groups: whether or not it is through assaults on women attending abortion clinics in the United States, the fountain of blood representing the 'martyrs' of the Iran–Iraq war, or suicide bombers against Israeli targets, the purveyors of 'true' religion have frequently demonstrated that preservation of human life is not their main concern. In the face of all this, liberalism looks like a fragile set of values.

Of women and children

Amongst the most prominent features of fundamentalism is its gender politics. Fundamentalist cultures are concerned with their own preservation and reproduction, hence with fertility and with the socialization process. Responsibility for this resides in religious leaders and in fathers, but women's adherence to communal values and practices is crucial. Most of the mechanisms of social control are directed at women, who represent the measure of the community's cohesion. If one wanted to be a structuralist in this morass, it would be easy: woman as the signifier passed around in the system, making it work. The letter of the law applies to her. Women are the property not only of the individual man, the father or husband, but of the community; in important ways, they are what power acts upon.[3] Injunctions concerning modesty apply predominantly to women, whose very existence threatens, through the power of sensuality, to make the fundamentalist edifice crumble. Women's voices should not be heard, for they distract the man from Torah; women are impure, so cannot be in holy places with men; women must be hidden, must keep out of the light. It does not need a full-blown Foucauldian analysis to reveal that in this machinery of repression there is fascination with sex, with its disruptive, energic capabilities, with its offer of something other than absolute obedience. Women represent this otherness in the heart of fundamentalism, a contaminating germ. The discourse being drawn upon here is the familiar one of bodily, worldly, feminine temptation ranged against masculine spirituality. Desexualizing women purifies the community, locating temptation and sexual excitement outside it, leaving the field clear for fantasies of the ideal. Regulating women symbolically and actually regulates the generative power of the community as a whole.[4]

To the extent that modernism has failed in its venture, it is because the belief in the power of rationality has been shown to be too simple and also too available to colonization by interest groups, in the service of patriarchy, imperialism and racism, for example. The breakdown of modernity allows irrationality and emotion back in, a process to be welcomed to the extent that it promotes the democratization of claims to knowledge, power and identity. But this also allows in irrational movements, from spiritualism and 'New Age-ism' to the fundamentalists I have been discussing. It is too simple to say, in this context, that fundamentalism offers an answer to the problem of finding an identity in a shifting world, although there is some truth in this formulation. It is more complete to say that it offers a way of riding the whirlwind. Like other ways of repudiating modernity, it is narcissistic in the psychoanalytic sense, being based on omnipotent fantasies and on the denial of otherness, of the existence of legitimate contradiction, and of alternative ways of being. It offers solace to lost souls, ways of succeeding in a world where the forces seem ranged against one, an easily accessible terrain of meaning and value, translated into the language of 'purity' and truth. Most of all, if one can accede to its regulating force, it offers release from the pain of uncertainty. In gender terms, it is as if the awesome power of the punitive father is used as a protection against the persecutory inner world, creating a 'maternal' space of community and security. That this maternal space is preserved only by vigorous and often vicious policing is part of its appeal, because the effectiveness of the policing attests to the continuing vigour of the father – and hence of the structure itself. Battling to keep the community pure, the fundamentalist 'father' may use the utmost brutality against enemies from without and within. Even if one does not like the Oedipal terms in which I have cast this drama, the way in which the adherents of fundamentalism draw strength from their movements' aggressive stances towards the world is worthy of note and anxious contemplation.

Into this maelstrom come children. The various tensions here involve the active wish of parents of all kinds to transmit something of their own allegiances – their identities – to their children measured against a set of liberal values which emphasize the freedom of every individual to make some kind of choice. Apart from the general difficulty that this choice is always constrained at least by the social forces which give it its context, there is the additional and specific problem that the fundamentalist cultures to which I am referring do not recognize the legitimacy of 'choice', let alone of liberal values. Indeed, each framework is in part built around the repudiation of the other through a process of scrutiny, judgement and ostracism. Liberals refute the authoritarianism of fundamentalism either as something 'primitive' or – as I have been doing – as an understandable but pernicious defensiveness; fundamentalists reject the secular, pluralistic, fragile morality of the West, which so often fails to provide any sense of rootedness. Faced with the choice for our children's development between a strong identity with clear moral purpose and sense of communal belonging and the characteristic anomie of late twentieth-century drift, who is to say for sure that a bit of totalitarian ideology is definitely wrong? Are we so certain that the rigidity of fundamentalist belief is antagonistic to mental health? Even in areas where it seems quite obvious that this is so, for example in sexual repressiveness and the subjugation of women, there are many speaking from within fundamentalist communities who claim otherwise. More generally, how does one pass on an identity constructed around doubt? If I want my children to have a strong identity as Jews, can I give it to them by opening out a debate about whether this is a good thing or not? On the other hand, what happens if they do not have this debate with themselves, with me as a parent, with the wider community? It might seem obvious that a fundamentalist community's failure to educate a child so that she or he has the widest possible capacity to choose between the array of careers and lifestyles on offer in the West is a constraint on freedom; but is there not a similar loss of freedom when one does not instil in a child the religious and communal values which are part of her or his family tradition? How easily can one 'choose' to join a community for which one does not have a deep, lived appreciation? Could I, when my children are seventeen or eighteen, say to them, 'I have not taught you anything, but now you are free to become whatever you like'?

These questions are themselves couched at something of the 'wrong' level for addressing the fundamentalist challenge. They take as their starting point the liberal concern with the development of the individual – with giving the growing child a sense of security, rootedness,

values and community. Whilst this is indeed a major interest of fundamentalist and other religious orders, it does not derive wholly from
concern for the well-being of the individual child. Rather, as all the
material discussed so far in this chapter should make obvious, it arises
out of the priority given to the preservation of the community and its
values.[5] The child's individual rights to self-determination may be
respected at the extreme, in the sense that she or he can usually choose
to cut themselves off from their community. But they are not accepted
as a *principle*, because the individual human subject is not the basic
unit of the moral order. The community, and, behind it, the religious
truth inscribed in its texts and authorities, is more primary, more
'fundamental'. Whilst most religious cultures allow specific laws to be
transgressed in order to save life, they do not organize themselves to
promote individual development or happiness, but to maintain order
and tradition. As Ilan Katz discusses in Chapter 6 in this book, the
continuing debate about whether circumcision is justifiable or not
exemplifies this issue. Whether circumcision is brutal and painful is
not the main point – in fact, it may even be desirable that it does cause
pain, because the important act is the subjugation of the individual
child to the community's commands, the explicit privileging of
bearing the yoke of responsibility for maintaining the tradition over
any individual child's (or parent's) preference.

The idea that the community's needs and entitlements might take
precedence over those of the individual child is a considerable challenge to the view of liberal moralists that places the rights of the
individual at the centre of moral systems. Indeed, in the classic 'rights
versus duties' tension of citizenship, fundamentalists quite straightfor-
wardly privilege duties: the 'best interests of the child' are less
significant than the best interests of the community. Clearly it can
often be argued that these two things go together (it is in the 'best
interests of the child' to be acceptable to the community), but this is
not always the case. Under the latter circumstances, preservation of the
community and its traditional religious values is of paramount concern
in fundamentalist cultures – passing down the truth to the next generation. One thing which it is very important to note here is that while
this privileging of the community occurs particularly strongly in totalitarian, authoritarian systems (of which religious fundamentalism is
the most vibrant contemporary example), it cannot be dismissed a
priori as an irrational or pernicious occurrence. All religious and most
other communities have the continuity of their culture as a central
concern. Nevertheless, the differences in the degree to which the
wishes and welfare of individuals can be subjugated to the moral prior-

ities of the community as a whole is an important marker of the distinction between fundamentalist and liberal cultures. To take a religious text as an example here, one of the founding stories of Judaism (Genesis 22) has Abraham prepared to sacrifice his son should God demand it; the fact that God does not in the end require this of him is a saving feature of the story to liberal eyes and has been encoded in the reading given it by mainstream orthodox Judaism. This makes the 'binding' of Isaac into both a test of Abraham's faith and a lesson against child sacrifice – the knife is stopped in mid-strike, human life is of paramount concern. Nevertheless, Abraham's readiness to give up his son in order to attest his obedience to God is the most striking and memorable aspect of the tale. Fundamentalist leaders, like Abraham before he is stopped, might not step back from the demand that children are sacrificed in the interests of the social-religious order, as many recent examples show, and in so doing they reveal their extremism. Liberal cultures make all absolute sacrifices of children illegitimate (even wartime offers only partial exceptions to this point), although, with definitions in child protection being as variable as they are (see Ilan Katz, Chapter 6, and David Archard, Chapter 5, this volume), it is not always certain that children's welfare is consistently put above that of the surrounding culture.

We have grown used, in the West, to a notion of childhood as an extended period for self-development, in which children have the right to explore alternative ways of being from within a protected context. By the end of this period they are supposed to have some notion of 'who they are', some sense of identity or identities. Fundamentalism reveals very clearly the potential vacuum which can arise here: values cannot usually simply be told to a child, they have to be *lived*. If the values of the community into which the child is born happen to emphasize subservience to religious truth, liberalism finds itself in a bind – unable to say, 'the child comes first', because that could be read as a racist disparagement of her or his culture (and anyway, what does that mean if 'coming first' should exclude the child from the culture – circumcision or arranged marriages being good examples?); but also unable to give up its own cultural set, its focus on the needs of the individual child as the most significant developmental value. Fundamentalism in this sense is truly liberalism's 'Other', revealing its boundary conditions and demanding that it recognizes that many communities do not place the individual child first, but instead have as their primary aim the preservation of their cultural beliefs and traditions.

Conclusion

Amongst the many challenges posed by fundamentalism in this area of 'moral agendas' and childhood, the main one seems to me to be how to find a way of constructing a critique which appreciates the intensity of a religious community's desire to maintain itself (and hence to socialize its children in specific ways) but which does not then buy into the fundamentalist demand that everything should be subservient to unquestionable and repressive religious authority. I have already noted the failure of multiculturalism to offer much of a way forward here. Looking for mechanisms through which different cultural groups can be recognized, multiculturalism has often accepted definitions of culture and community offered by religious and political leaders affiliated to fundamentalist groups, because they make the most vociferous and coherent claims. Policing the boundaries of their communities, they can be seen clearly by those on the outside; they also speak a language of ethnic identity and equal rights congruent with neo-liberalism. Anti-racism as a political movement, at least in Britain, has also had terrible problems, as the constant shifting of preferred terms to deal with the multiplicity of positions represented in the word 'black' testifies ('black', 'Black', 'black and Asian', 'ethnic minority', 'minority ethnic', 'ethnically diverse', etc.). Both these movements have been more concerned with the boundaries between communities than with the internal politics of those communities themselves; they have also tended to hold firm, sometimes rigid and occasionally authoritarian views themselves about what is right politically and culturally. As such, they have too often failed to hear and support dissenting voices – surely the only position from which a genuine counter-practice can begin.

Postmodernism, as an alternative response to the contradictions of modernism, is too intellectual and too incoherent for everyday practice, although it does offer important insights in its celebration of 'difference' (which could be a method of opposing fundamentalist certainties) and more innovatively in its recognition of the place of the irrational in fixing meaning. This includes the idea, for example, that investment in an ideology is neither 'false consciousness' nor purely rational self-seeking, but holds within it a response to the anxiety generated by what has come to be known in Lacanian circles as the Real, the unanalysable aspect of experience that crouches always at the margins of awareness (see Žižek, 1991). It is exactly this aspect of experience – including all those regions of unpredictability listed earlier – that terrorizes people into seeking out safe havens within which thinking can be closed down. Fundamentalism, therefore, is not just a *defence against* the anxiety produced by modern life, it is also energized *by* this anxiety – it is a *modern* phenomenon – and its complexity and power derive as much from what it apparently fears as from what it offers. Facing the Real, acknowledging and working with the anxiety it produces, is something that our politics have to begin to do if fundamentalist and other totalitarian world-views are to be opposed. This means creating modes of work that do not reduce experience to 'narratives' and do not romanticize cultural stories as if they were innocent and timeless kernels from which purposeful engagement with the world necessarily arises. Rather, willingness to own a set of unapologetic and not very relativistic ethical values – in the same way as has characterized feminism's stance in other areas connected with gender and abuse – is a necessary component of anti-fundamentalist practice.

More pragmatically, I have drawn attention here to the difficulties produced by seeing things from the outside. Faced with fundamentalism, outsiders tend to repudiate it or embrace its exoticism; it is harder to see how it misrepresents the complexity and diversity of the traditions upon which it draws. Oppositional practices have to be built on knowledge, on an extension of anti-racism, to allow expression of the voices of oppressed groups from within minorities. Almost always, given the misogyny present in most (if not all) fundamentalist world-views, this will involve gender politics. It will require recognition of the variety of religious and cultural groupings, and it will also require seeking out and forming alliances with dissenting voices within religious communities and recruiting them into political work. This is not necessarily a colonizing enterprise on the part of liberalism. Part of the problem is that liberalism too easily grants fundamentalists the right to speak on behalf of people who do not necessarily share their views, even though they remain attached in many ways to their culture, community and religious practices. Rather, recognizing the importance of taking a moral or an ethical stance, however 'culturally specific' it might be argued to be, could allow articulation of the real dilemmas involved in balancing individuals' rights – such as the issue of the 'best interests of the child' – against communal requirements. More forcefully, anti-fundamentalist activity which nevertheless acknowledges the legitimacy of religious and cultural perspectives in forging children's developmental contexts could enhance the capacity of members of religious and cultural groupings to draw on the life-affirming aspects of their heritage. There always will be tension between 'revealed' religion and the liberal impulse, but for those who participate in religious practices this does not feel like a tension which can only be resolved through either fundamentalism or repudiation of religion in its entirety. This is probably because religious affiliation is concerned with much more than belief: as argued throughout this chapter, it is fuelled by identifications with cultural, political and historical patterns that define the sense of community in which personal identity has some of its most compelling roots. The fundamentalist appropriation of this complex pattern of identification is one of its most pernicious aspects. Exposing and counteracting the pull of fundamentalism is consequently a vital task for political and moral activity from within and without.

Notes

1 This chapter is adapted from an article entitled 'Fundamentalism, gender and family therapy' which appeared in the *Journal of Family Therapy* 19, 417–30, 1997.
2 Ilan Katz's discussion of the difficulties generated by notions of 'cultural sensitivity' (see Chapter 6, this volume) clearly shows the ways in which apparently anti-oppressive practice can confirm the construction of members of 'minority' groups as 'others'. One manifestation of this is the failure of the 'cultural sensitivity' position to engage with the complexity and heterogeneity of the world-views of the cultures under inspection.
3 This is one obvious place where the political links between fundamentalism and nationalism become apparent. In nationalism, women are usually positioned as 'bearers of the nation', often idealized and desexualized (or contrasted with the 'bad woman' of the other nation), but symbolically representing that-which-must-be-preserved. Women who do not want to be pure and ideal in this way risk the nation's retributive wrath. For an influential case example of this, see Theweleit (1977).
4 When I read this passage to some members of my community, some of the women said that it felt completely untrue to their experience. For them, the separation of male and female worlds represented an area of the preservation of feminine life, away from the demeaning structures of masculine discourse, and hence an arena of self-empowerment and satisfaction. Others have noted that within fundamentalist communities the sense of security and value women gain from their connection with other women can more than make up for the apparent loss of freedom. However, the *regulation* of femininity under these conditions is very stringent; dissenting lifestyles are not easily achieved by women who do not wish to be part of the fundamentalist order.
5 In the discussion following this paper at the Moral Agendas workshop, Ilan Katz described some research on the mental health provision needed by members of a traditional Muslim community in Britain. He noted that the premises of the study were in some ways alien to the community involved. The parents

saw things purely in moral terms....In other words what they saw was that their children were misbehaving. Their responsibility as parents was to ensure that their children continued the Muslim religion. That was their primary responsibility. It was not a responsibility to their children as individual people. Therefore the idea that they had done something wrong as parents which created misbehaviour did not enter into it. Their responsibility was not to behave nicely to their children so that their children were happy. Their responsibility was to ensure that their children carried on the tradition. And if this involved sending their children back to Pakistan or getting their child married at the age of twelve or thirteen, then they would do that.

13 Failing children

Responding to young people with 'behavioural difficulties'

Daniel Monk

The behaviour of children increasingly poses problems for governments. The belief, however sincere, that their behaviour is problematic and a legitimate object of concern, reflects and serves to uphold childhood as a social category of enduring cultural and practical significance for policy-makers in modern Western societies. A variety of calculations and perceptions give rise to the conceptualization of child behaviour as a growing problem. They include, for example: concerns regarding educational standards and the need for an educated workforce (Department for Education and Employment [DfEE], 1997) and moral panics in response to an assumed increase in criminality and immorality amongst young people. These concerns and perceptions translate into a plethora of statutory provisions, programmes and practices. Identifying and examining these attempts to govern children reinforces Nikolas Rose's much-quoted observation that 'Childhood is the most intensely governed sector of personal existence'[1] (Rose, 1989). Underlying these perceptions are complex and more fluid anxieties regarding the nature and function of the concept of youth (Jenks, 1996; James and Prout, 1997; Wyn and White, 1997). Yet, significantly, the acknowledgement of the contingency of childhood often presents a challenge to and for public and policy responses to the problems, and indeed problematizations, of aspects of childhood; for the perception that the behaviour of large numbers of children constitutes a problem is often characterized as an unquestionable common sense 'truth' and one that justifies, demands and requires a solution.

The desire to intervene and manage the problems of childhood is reflected in law by an ever-increasing number of legal constructions of problematized children. Most recently the Education Act 1997 introduced, uncontroversially, the new category of children with 'behavioural difficulties'[2] (Monk, 1997). Also within education law we find 'excluded children'[3] and 'children with special educational needs'[4] and, for example, in civil child law the 'Gillick competent child'[5], children 'in care'[6] and the much wider category of 'children in need'.[7] These legal objects represent not so much 'real' children but semantic artifacts (King and Piper, 1995) or contingent constructs (O'Donovan, 1993, p. 90), which operate within clearly defined statutory and professional frameworks (see Alison Diduck, Chapter 8, this volume). Consequently, while they are not mutually exclusive, and indeed children very often wear more than one of these masks or labels, within each category or framework the child's conduct is explained, and responded to, in distinct, often conflicting ways.

The new category of children with behavioural difficulties is not defined by statute, but the provisions indicate that it includes excluded children and children with special educational needs (Monk, 1997). It is these two constructions that form the focus of this chapter. Before examining each of these constructions in turn it is important to acknowledge that they are not just legal but *educational* responses to child behaviour, and that this is therefore quite a narrow focus and excludes reference to civil child care law or the criminal juvenile justice system. Education law and child care law differ significantly, particularly with regard to children's rights (Bainham, 1988, 1996; Harris, 1993a; Jeffs, 1995; Freeman, 1996); consequently, while talking about excluded children and children with special educational needs, it is perhaps more appropriate to talk of *pupils* rather than *children* to indicate that these are quite distinct social categories, that they are located within distinct institutions (the school and the family), and that the problematizations of the behaviour and attainments of the young people within these categories are contingent on distinct discursive understandings.

The aim here is not to criticize educational and legal responses from a particular ideological or functional perspective but, rather 1) to trace the contingent nature of these responses from critical theoretical perspectives; 2) to reveal the extent to which the problems which they endeavour to resolve are not simply those of individual children but of society and a particular social order; and, consequently, 3) to demonstrate the inevitable limits to claims that these responses can offer totalizing or universal understandings or solutions.

The 'excluded child'

The number of children permanently excluded from school in the United Kingdom has risen from just under 3,000 in the years 1990–1 to over 13,000 in 1996 (Berridge and Brodie, 1997). This dramatic increase has been perceived as a matter of concern by a variety of legal, educational and child welfare commentators, and as a problem that requires government attention and action (Brodie, 1995; Children's Legal Centre, 1996; Childright, 1996; Parsons, 1996; Brereton, 1997; Sinclair, 1997).

Numerous explanations exist for the increase and these generally fall into one of two broad categories. Within the first category the rise in exclusions and associated discipline problems within schools are understood as an indication of increasing antisocial behaviour by children. Consequently, the focus of this category is on the factors that are perceived to influence the behaviour of individual children, such as lack of parental responsibility; misguided progressive teaching methods; the bad example set by teachers striking and wearing inappropriate clothes; increased violence on television; the condition of school buildings; failure to recognize and resource special educational needs; and underlying structural inequalities in society.[8] These explanatory factors, identified by academics, journalists and politicians, often reflect a particular political or ideological view of society and, consequently, serve to justify a range of often conflicting programmes and policies.

The second category challenges the assumption that the rise reflects changing behaviour amongst children. Exponents of this approach argue, most plausibly, that it simply 'is not feasible that children's behaviour could have deteriorated so much within so short a space of time' (Berridge and Brodie, 1997, p. 5). Instead they argue that the increase is directly connected to the radical changes in the organization of the educational system over the last fifteen years, in particular the introduction, through various provisions, of a market-based system which 'creates winners and losers…and acts against those problematic and underachieving pupils who are expensive to educate' (*ibid.*). These policies serve to problematize pupil behaviour not solely on the basis of discipline or manageability but also on account of their effect on the school in league tables and allocation of resources (Carvel, 1997; Brodie, 1995).

Underlying this more critical approach is an appreciation of the fact that the problematization of children's behaviour which results in exclusion is not a simple response to 'reality', but rather involves, and indeed is contingent upon, shifting constructions of the good or ideal pupil as well as the purpose of education against which the appropriateness of a child's behaviour can be evaluated and judged. An advantage of this approach is its ability to explain, although only in part, why it is that the vast majority of excluded children are boys

(Brodie, 1995); for it is girls that are now increasingly perceived as generally behaving in the ideal manner required of pupils (Tyler, 1997).

Despite these complex and conflicting political and social explanations underlying the rise in school exclusions, the 'excluded child', within the context of individual school exclusion proceedings is a relatively simple construct; in particular issues of gender, class and race, which have significant implications in the practice of exclusions, are overlooked and deemed irrelevant. This process of simplification and individualization is made possible through the perceiving or interpreting of the conduct of the excluded child in quasi-criminal terms (King and Piper, 1995, p. 104), a process which serves to construct the excluded child as morally 'bad'. Within this model the school represents a miniature society in which the head teacher, supported by the governing body, is the law maker, and the standards, or rules, of behaviour which they determine represent the criminal law of that society and the excluded child, a criminal.

This model is upheld by statute, which determines that the power to exclude pupils is exercisable only by a head teacher,[9] and by the Department for Education and Employment (DfEE) guidance circular, which states that, 'Exclusion is a disciplinary sanction to be used...only in response to serious breaches of a school's policy on behaviour or criminal law' (DfEE, 1994d, Circular 10/94, para 2). Similarly, where the decision to exclude a pupil or to reinstate an excluded pupil is subsequently challenged and brought before a school's appeal committee, it is the disruptive or inappropriate behaviour of the pupil, the 'unlawful conduct', as opposed to other aspects of the pupil or the school itself, that forms the central focus for consideration. While appeal committees have a wide degree of discretion,[10] they are not obliged by statute to consider the interests of any of the parties involved when they 'decide that the pupil in question was not guilty of the conduct which the Head Teacher relied on as grounds for his permanent exclusion'.[11] When this is not the case the committee must have regard to the disciplinary measures publicized by the head teacher[12] in order to establish whether or not the excluded child's behaviour breaches the 'standard of behaviour which is to be regarded as acceptable'.[13] In this way, the binary distinction good pupil/bad pupil is reproduced within the realm of a legal discourse and the legal framework which lays down the procedures and considers the evidence according to which such judgements may be made.

However, in addition to this emphasis on the behaviour of the pupil, as opposed to the pupil him or herself, appeal committees are also obliged by statute to have regard to the interests of the pupil, as well as the interests of the other pupils at the school and the members of staff.[14] Similarly, the Department for Education and Employment guidance encourages appeal committees to have regard to other information regarding the excluded child, such as the possibility of the pupil having a special educational need and the domestic circumstances of the child (DfEE, 1994d, Circular 10/94, paras 5, 6). However, despite these attempts to broaden the focus of appeal committees, it is suggested that the interests of the child are rarely a crucial consideration in exclusion decisions. Indeed, the fact that the consequences of exclusion for many excluded pupils are inadequate, part-time education and increased vulnerability to involvement in crime (Berridge and Brodie, 1997, p. 2; Hayden, 1994; Parsons, 1996; Childright, 1996; Audit Commission, 1996) suggests that exclusion is rarely, if ever, in a child's best interests. Rather, while other factors relating to an excluded child may be considered, within the quasi-criminal model they are marginalized and, as King and Piper suggest in the context of juvenile justice, are only relevant to the extent that they demonstrate the pupil's 'dangerousness' to society (in this context the school) and degree of moral responsibility (King and Piper, 1995, p. 104). This interpretation is supported, albeit unintentionally, by the Department for Education and Employment guidance circular itself; for the circular advises schools that assessing whether reinstatement of an excluded pupil would be 'seriously detrimental to the education or welfare of the pupil' is a criterion which provides not, as one might expect, a test to establish whether or not exclusion would be in the best interest of the pupil but, rather, 'a test to assist in distinguishing between serious and minor offences' (DfEE, 1994d, Circular 10/94 paras 5, 6). This demonstrates clearly how information from educational and welfare discourses, far from opening up the legal discourse to other more complex perceptions about a pupil's conduct, and far from being used to establish what the effects of exclusion will be, is rather reconstituted within the quasi-criminal law system for exclusions in a way that reduces the complexities of the situation to a hybrid moral/legal communication.

In a variety of other legal contexts, social welfare and educational factors relating to children are perceived and utilized in quite a different way. This is particularly significant in the context of excluded children as they are very rarely *only* excluded children. In fact, large numbers of them are 'children in care', 'children in need', 'children with special educational needs' and young offenders (Brodie, 1995;

Department of Health and Social Services Inspectorate/OFSTED, 1995; Audit Commission, 1996; Sinclair, 1997).

Child care proceedings, under the Children Act 1989, present an interesting contrast to exclusions and, in particular, highlight the fluid and complex relationship between professional, or systematic, discourses and individual responses. In the case of exclusions, it is not lawyers or the judiciary, but the head teacher, school governors and appeal committees who determine the issue of whether a pupil's conduct is acceptable or unacceptable, 'legal' or 'illegal'. Despite the legalistic nature of school exclusion proceedings, when the decisions of exclusion appeal committees are reviewed by the courts, the judiciary generally limit their review to issues of procedural fairness (Harris, 1997b; Harris and Parsons, 1998; Monk, 1997). In a recent case, while the court held that the decision to exclude was quasi-judicial and not administrative in character, it refused to address the merits of the decision, in this case a refusal to reinstate, on the basis that 'educational factors were outside the provenance of the court'.[15] In contrast, in child care proceedings welfare considerations, which include educational factors, albeit reconstituted within legal discourse, are central concerns of judges and lawyers. This contrast between care proceedings and exclusion appeals indicates that legal discourse may occur outside of the courts and lawyers' chambers and that, conversely, the courts are not impervious to other discourses, which is to say that the legal discourse is not confined to geographical or institutional locations and that there is a distinction between legal domain and legal discourse[16] (King and Piper, 1995, p. 106).

School exclusions are explicitly described by statute and government guidance as being a form of punishment and implicit in the quasi-criminal nature of punishment by exclusion is the construction of the excluded child as having a degree of culpability for his or her conduct. In the United Kingdom, while the possibility that the child has a special educational need or troubled domestic circumstances may be considered, it is no defence, the central focus in exclusion proceedings being *the conduct of the pupil*.

In contrast, in the United States if a child is suspended or excluded for violating disciplinary rules and is punished because of his or her disability related behaviour, suspension for more than ten days per year is illegal. However an important proviso to this is that it must be the *child's disability that caused the behaviour* and, significantly, learning and behavioural problems that result from environmental or cultural reasons or economic disadvantage are specifically excluded from the definition of disability[17] (Weisz, 1995, p. 198). An important implication of this, which applies by default in the United Kingdom, is that, in the context of school exclusions, lack of responsible parenting in no way reduces a pupil's culpability. This is perhaps surprising in light of the fact that pupils have no independent rights in exclusion appeals and that the 'relevant person' in these proceedings, who is subsequently entitled to make representations, is defined in law as the parent when the pupil is under the age of eighteen.[18]

However, the notion of culpability as a characteristic of the excluded child demonstrates a crucial distinction between punishment and forms of treatment such as special educational needs. Hobbes wrote that "'tis against the law of nature to punish the innocent' (OED). Innocence is a characteristic of great importance in many social and cultural conceptualizations of childhood (Archard, 1993, pp. 37–8; Jenks, 1996). The excluded child, through his or her demonstrative and proven guilty conduct, is not an innocent child. Consequently the excluded child is not only excluded from school but to a certain extent from the social category of childhood itself. In this respect, the excluded child is similar to the sexual child – pregnant teenage pupils are also removed from classrooms partly because their presence challenges and destabilizes the idealized norm of children as sexual innocents (Monk, 1998). As Jenks comments, in connection with the media responses to the Bulger trial, 'by refusing children who commit acts of violence acceptance within the category of child, the public was reaffirming to itself the essence of what children are' and that 'the system of classification stays intact by resisting the "defilement" of the abhorrent case' (Jenks, 1996, p. 129).

However, there are problems with this analysis. In particular the belief, and policy, of successive governments that firm discipline is necessary for all pupils suggests that childhood innocence, at least in the context of education, has less significance than the diametrically opposite construction of the child as originally and innately sinful. Nevertheless, because the excluded child fails to act in accordance with the school's acceptable standards of behaviour and fails to respond to school discipline, the child is excluded, not necessarily from childhood but, more precisely, from the educational and social category of 'pupil'.

During the debates in the UK parliament concerning the Education Act 1997, the Bill, as it then was, was criticized for introducing the term 'disqualified persons' to refer to pupils permanently excluded from more than two schools.[19] While the expression was removed from the Act, the provision, which gives schools the right to refuse admission to such children, remained unchanged.[20] The expression 'disqualified persons' is, however, significant and apposite, in that children excluded from more than one school are indeed disqualified to the extent that they are rendered unfit or unable to be a 'pupil'. Furthermore, the term 'disqualified *persons*' was used as opposed to 'disqualified *children*', which again signifies that as regards education they have lost the privileges and obligations that society owed to them when they were characterized as 'children' and have hence become legal 'persons'. This has a practical significance because many children within this category are close to the age threshold of sixteen, up to which they are entitled to education; in effect the provision repositions them over this threshold in order that their biological age more closely reflects their social status, which is to say that despite being under the age of sixteen they are no longer entitled to education. The expression was replaced in the Act by the term 'children'. This was in response to concerns that the word 'disqualified' suggested that the state could indeed in some way abdicate its responsibilities to certain children, that it would in effect label these children as being 'beyond hope', and that this was dangerous for society as well as being damaging for the children concerned.[21] Relabelling them in this way reflected not simply a humane and liberal amendment to the Act, but also a desire to salvage the characterization of these individuals as children and, consequently, as future adults and citizens – therefore as legitimate 'objects of concern' – in order to legitimize and encourage alternative responses to their behaviour, so protecting the future social order.

Discipline, in the context of exclusions, consequently takes on a double meaning: it refers first to schools' repressive, juridical system of punishment; and second, to the power/knowledge schema whereby schools represent a privileged location for policing and establishing the boundaries between normal and abnormal pupil behaviour (McGillivray, 1997, p. 4) and between the categories of 'pupil' and 'adult'. Put another way, discipline represents two processes: that which keeps the pupil present before the knowledge, and that which establishes knowledge of the pupil (Hoskin, 1990).

Underlying these practices are conflicts within society as to how children who do not conform to idealized conceptualizations of 'child' or 'pupil' should be treated. Inherent within these conflicts are deeper concerns and anxieties about the meaning of childhood and its relationship with the social order of the future. That this is particularly clear in the context of education is in part due to the fact that education, as a form of social policy, has an explicitly aspirational role, one of its clear functions being the construction of future adults (Finch, 1984). This contrasts with child care law's emphasis on the protection of children.

The child with 'special educational needs'

Alongside the dramatic rise in school exclusions there has been the development of programmes and a new legal framework for children with special educational needs (Riddell and Brown, 1994; Wedell, 1990; Harris, 1997a). Having until recently played a relatively marginalized role, over a short space of time special educational needs have become a legitimate and influential factor in all policies regarding children's social and educational development and welfare (Audit Commission, 1992; DfEE, 1997). It is perhaps informative to talk of the 'discovery of special educational needs', which bears certain similarities to the 'discovery' of child sexual abuse (Parton, 1985), as a means to understanding the conditions of possibility underlying the increase in public and political concern and the growth of the special educational needs industry. This helps us to appreciate how these developments reflect not simply a progressive welfare-based agenda but more complex power relations, changing perceptions of problematic children and the definitions of educational failure (Barton and Oliver, 1997).

Special educational need can be perceived as a 'soft' welfaristic response to children with behavioural difficulties, a response which serves to 'correct the rigours of the school' (McGillivray, 1997, p. 4). Central to this characterization is the fact that it is blame free; consequently, the child with a special educational need is constructed as 'ill' and in need of special treatment, as opposed to being 'bad' and in need of punishment. From a Foucauldian perspective this represents not just a humane and progressive response, but also another schema of power/knowledge – an alternative disciplinary process for the governing of pupils (Hunter, 1996; Rose, 1996). This approach allows programmes for special educational needs to be understood as a modern technique of government, which, in contrast to the juridical system of punishment, tries to enable those pupils whose behaviour has been problematized to perform in accordance with a set of normative calculations as to what is appropriate behaviour. It does not suggest that special educational needs programmes are necessarily negative or that they conflict with children's welfare. Rather, it challenges a perception of them as programmes for the achievement of self-realization (Hunter, 1996), which is to say that in the problematizing of certain pupils' behaviour and in the establishing of the ideal norm for pupils, programmes for special educational needs are not simply a response to individual need, but are the result of a complex interaction of social, cultural and economic calculations and interests.

Consequently, special educational needs are not solely or primarily the needs of the pupil (Tomlinson, 1981; Barton and Tomlinson, 1984; Barton and Oliver, 1997).

The discursive origins of special educational needs can be identified clearly in the scientific discipline of developmental psychology (Bart, 1984). Within this discipline, and in particular as a result of the influence of Piaget's work, child development and learning are conceptualized as natural processes in which children acquire cognitive competencies according to universal and stratified sequences based largely on age (Jenks, 1996, p. 23; Sutton, 1981). This 'ideology of development' constructs boundaries between the social categories of adult and child and implicitly equates adult intelligence with a neutral scientific rationality. Critical analyses of these theories highlight how within this ideology, 'the development of thought is indifferent to the actual content of thought' (Venn and Walkerine, quoted in Jenks, 1996, p. 25) and that, as Jenks describes, 'real children are subjected to the violence of a contemporary mode of scientific rationality which reproduces itself at the expense of their difference' (Jenks, 1996, p. 25).

These critical analyses of developmental psychology can equally be applied to the legal definition and construction of special educational needs. The Education Act 1996 defines special educational needs as a 'learning difficulty which calls for special educational provision'. A child is defined by the Act as having a learning difficulty in the following three ways:

(a) a greater difficulty in learning than the majority of children of his age; or
(b) a disability which either prevents or hinders him from making use of educational facilities of a kind generally provided for children of his age (in schools within the area of the LEA); or
(c) if under the age of five a child would have a Special Educational Need by the time he reaches school age unless special provision is made.[22]

Within all the above categories the assessment of special educational needs is dependent on the identification of what is normal for a child of a particular age. Yet these norms, established through detailed surveillance of children in clinics and schools represent little more than 'a standard based upon the average abilities or performances of children of a certain age in a particular task or a specified ability' (Rose, 1989, p. 142). The importance attached to the ability to ascertain the truth of the normal child upholds the ideology of development and ensures that in the context of special educational need the desirability of difference is highly problematic (Barton and Tomlinson, 1984; Barton and Oliver, 1997). Indeed, while the government *Code of Practice on the Identification and Assessment of Special Educational Needs* acknowledges that *all* children may at some stage have a special educational need (DfEE, 1994a), the emphasis is on treatment as opposed to recognizing the challenge that behaviour which deviates from the norm presents for educators.

In practice, special educational needs are assessed, almost exclusively, by reading ability and, to a lesser extent, by mathematical skills; no-one is referred for an assessment for lack of interest or aptitude for art or sport. Consequently, it is not learning per se that is crucial in the diagnosis of a special educational need, but rather the ability to learn particular knowledge in a particular way. The marginalization of art in the curriculum is one example of how the system of education upholds a particular concept of ability by assessing intelligence in such a way that literal and scientific processes are more privileged than visual and conceptual mental processes (Robinson, 1995; Harland and Kinder, 1995; Barton and Oliver, 1997). As a result, as Galloway comments, 'whether a child's attainments or behaviour are seen as evidence of special educational needs depends on what parents, employers and government expect from the educational system' (Galloway *et al.*, 1994). In this way the seemingly neutral theories of educational psychology translated into programmes of special educational need can be seen to reinforce an educational ideology of vocationalism (Jenks, 1996).

The category of disability in the legal definition of special educational needs ensures that the diagnosis of a psychological disorder or syndrome is often crucial in the assessment of special educational needs. It legitimizes an influential role for experts in disputes (Harris, 1997a) and clearly reinforces the relationship between learning in school and scientific theories of child development. Psychological pathology confers a legitimacy on behaviour that deviates from the norm. However, it is a conditional legitimacy in that there is an implicit recognition that this is an undesirable state (Bart, 1984).

The disability category has become increasingly significant as a plethora of clinical disorders, such as dyslexia, are discovered and, once legitimized, are accepted as evidence of learning disability for the purposes of special educational needs. Significantly, these clinical understandings of children are not restricted to low achievers but also, for example, construct 'gifted' and 'exceptionally able' children as two clinically distinguished categories (Weisz, 1995; Lorenz, 1997). High-achieving children clearly challenge the norm and the adult/child divide. However, they are rarely identified as having special educational needs and this is not simply a matter of resources. Their 'difference' is not encouraged, but nor is it identified as a condition in need of treatment.

One consequence of the medical 'within-the child' construction of special educational needs is that historical and cultural factors are excluded from the assessment. For example, the ideal Victorian child that was seen and not heard could today quite possibly be perceived as withdrawn and suffering from a communication disorder; he or she would be treated and not praised.

An interesting example of a more recently discovered condition is the current 'epidemic' (Slee, 1995, p. 167) of attention deficit disorder (ADD). Diagnosis of ADD is dependent on a child displaying a number of behavioural attributes. These might include: often not appearing to listen when spoken to; often losing things such as pencils and school assignments; disliking tasks such as homework; running about in situations in which it is inappropriate; being easily distracted; leaving a classroom seat when being seated is expected; being noisy when taking part in quiet leisure activities (World Health Organization classification quoted in Silver, 1997). A controversial, but increasingly used, treatment of ADD is the drug Ritalin. This drug, a form of amphetamine which was initially developed as a slimming drug, is claimed by its proponents to stimulate the brain so that it has the paradoxical effect of calming down a child and enabling concentration. This practice clearly illustrates the extent to which social pathology is treated as individual illness, and demonstrates how medical knowledge and expertise operate as a legitimate technique of modern government (Rose, 1996; Tyler, 1997).

The Department for Education and Employment guidance circular regarding the education of children with 'emotional and behavioural difficulties', a category which includes ADD, acknowledges the fact that definitions of emotional and behavioural difficulties are extremely complex and that it can be argued that every child has an emotional and behavioural difficulty of some kind at some point in their development (DfEE, 1994c, Circular 9/94, para 1). However, it advises that the complex distinction between normal, but stressed behaviour, and behaviour arising from mental illness is important because 'each needs to be treated differently' (*ibid.*, para 2). Implicit within the notion of treatment here is the problematization of child behaviour that deviates from the norm.

The category in the legal definition of special education needs concerning the child under five indicates that one of the purposes of special educational needs is to prepare children for the move from nursery to school, a moment that marks the end of carefree childish games and the beginning of adult-like work in the form of a particular type of learning. The distinction between work and play, with the trivialization of the latter, is learnt at an early age and indicates the role that education has in preparing children for a particular social role (Sherman, 1997). Again, this challenges the individualistic, or 'within-the-child', and scientific conceptualization of special educational needs, for, in this context, it serves to 'assist' children in the transition from the social category of 'infant' to that of a 'pupil'.

Clearly then special educational need is not simply a self-contained product of a scientific discourse; rather, it is, by definition as well as in administration and practice, essentially a social, educational and political construction (Sutton, 1981; Barton and Tomlinson, 1984; Slee, 1995). As a result, while special educational need draws significantly on the construction of reality within scientific discourses, it exists independently of them. In the process which translates discourse into an education programme and the child with special educational needs into a legal construct, there is a necessary 'interference' between science and the discourses of education, law and politics. Indeed the increased legitimacy and importance attached to special educational need in recent years, and in particular its identification as a crucial factor in tackling the growing problem of child behaviour, has increasingly taken the concept of special educational needs away from the contained world of the clinic and into the public arena and political debate, as well as into schools and the courts.

A critical illustration of this process of reconstruction or 'interference' is the calculation of how widespread special educational needs are. Amongst educational psychologists there is little consensus, largely due to the lack of any clear definition. Research varies in its conclusions to such a degree that between 2 per cent and 60 per cent of pupils may at any one time be considered as having a special educational need (Galloway, 1994). However, in the context of government policy, following the recommendations of the Warnock Commission, the figure of 20 per cent has been established (Warnock, 1978; DfEE, 1997). The result, in practice, is that while information regarding the severity of a child's behaviour in the clinic is used to distinguish between one disorder and another, the same information in schools and Local Education Authorities is used to determine whether or not resources can justifiably be allocated to the child (Thomas and Davis,

1997) – or whether there may in fact be an easier or cheaper option, such as exclusion.

One consequence of this limited provision for special educational need is the fact that parents faced with the denial of access to special services increasingly challenge Local Education Authority decisions not to provide a statement that their child has a special educational need (Oliver and Austen, 1996; Harris, 1997b). The market-based reforms of the education system since 1979 have in a variety of ways constructed parents as consumers rather than passive recipients of services (Bash and Coulby, 1989; Harris, 1993a; Barron, 1996) and, together with greater central regulation, this has led to increased legalism within the education system (Harris, 1997b). This is particularly the case in the context of special educational need which is now the most litigated issue in education. The result of this interference between special educational need and legal discourse is that the complex medical and psychosocial issues surrounding the diagnosis of a child are dramatically simplified: the child is classified as a child either with or without a special educational need. In this way, the decision to statement a child may be expressed in the simple binary terms of needing/not needing special education.

Similarly, while the effect of and predictions regarding the possible outcome of treatment are crucial for educational psychologists, teachers and parents, within the legal discourse, if the child is over the age of five, the success or failure of treatment is a marginal concern in determining the central issue of whether or not a child has a special educational need.

Conclusion

In conclusion I make two interrelated but distinct points to demonstrate how critical theoretical approaches serve to illuminate and to a certain extent challenge current political and professional responses to pupil behaviour and attainments.

The first point is to emphasize the similarities between exclusions and special educational needs. This challenges the perception of them as oppositional practices reflecting the dichotomy of welfare and justice, similar to the dichotomy evident in political debates regarding juvenile crime. Welfare adherents argue that as the categorization of special educational needs addresses the causes of inappropriate child behaviour, increased resources for special educational needs, together with earlier intervention (Sandow, 1990), would result in a reduction in the need to resort to exclusions (DfEE, 1997). Conversely, others argue that it is stricter and more rigorously applied discipline that is required, with disruptive pupils being excluded quickly and for longer periods – a policy implicitly adopted in the Education Act 1997 (Hodgkin, 1997). However, the construction of this dichotomy, though it is relevant, obscures the fact that both exclusions and special educational needs serve a normative function. By this I mean that they are not only *responses* to inappropriate or abnormal pupil behaviour but that they both play a critical role in, and are an important site for, the construction and definition of the problem.

In the context of exclusions this is achieved through the assertion of acceptable standards of behaviour, and indeed the normative function of exclusion is explicit within the quasi-criminal structure of the system. In contrast, in the special educational needs system the norms are expressed through the neutral language of science, as opposed to the sovereign-like commands of a head teacher. This reflects the shift from repressive juridical control to more intimate and invasive techniques of government (Tyler, 1997; Rose, 1989, 1996). The fact that while parents generally challenge exclusions, they plead for special educational needs is itself indicative of this shift and of the invasiveness of this form of government as it demonstrates the internalization of the psy-disciplines. As Rose comments, 'The tension generated by the gap between normality and actuality bonds our personal projects inseparably to expertise' (Rose, 1989, p. 208).

This highlighting of the normative purpose of both exclusions and special educational needs challenges the perception of them as alternative solutions to the problem of aberrant children, precisely because they are both characterized as *solutions*. For implicit within this approach is a failure to incorporate an appreciation of the fact that the construction of the problem child is essential for the construction of the ideal or normal child. This approach explains why increased efforts to help, cure and solve the problem of abnormal children, as evident from the rise in exclusions and the increased role of special educational needs, have not resulted in a reduction in the number of such children, but rather the opposite. In a similar way the introduction of the National Curriculum, while raising the standard of education for many, has also resulted in the construction of what the leader of the head teachers' union referred to as 'an underclass of children' (Carvel, 1997).

The second concluding point utilizes Teubner's account of autopoietic (or self-referential systems) theory. This emphasizes not only the similarities between special educational needs and exclusions but also the differences between them. This approach is notably different from that described in the first point, above, in that it focuses not on the oppressive and disciplinary nature of special educational needs and exclusions but rather characterizes them as systems of communication. King and Piper have demonstrated how this approach challenges the welfare/justice dichotomy (King and Piper, 1995, p. 11), but of particular relevance in this context is the critique it presents to the suggestion, frequently made, that closer collaboration and communication between the relevant professionals and agencies will result in, and are necessary for, a more 'child-centred approach' (DfEE Circular 1994b, Circular 8/94; Sinclair, 1997).

As legal constructs, the excluded child and the child with special educational needs both simplify, individualize and depoliticize complex issues. This serves to marginalize and overlook the significant implications of gender, race and class in the composition of the children within these categories (Barton and Oliver, 1997). Similarly, while factors such as bad or inappropriate teaching and failing schools, as opposed to failing pupils, are identified as crucial factors in understanding the conduct and attainments of pupils (Elton, 1989), and indeed are high on the political agenda (DfEE, 1997), in the legal construction of the excluded child and the child with special educational needs these factors are deemed irrelevant. Furthermore, the possibly uninspiring and rigid nature of the curriculum is never a relevant factor in explaining the lack of interest or aptitude of a pupil, in the context of special educational needs, or in explaining the disruptive behaviour of a pupil, in the context of exclusions (Russell, 1990; Visser, 1993).

Both those children who are excluded and those with special educational needs represent political constructs of otherwise ill-defined and unspecific behaviours. In both cases their construction is the result of the political system confronting perturbations in its environment arising from the constructions of other discourses. In the case of special educational needs the external discourse is predominantly that of educational psychology; in the case of school exclusions it is predominantly that of morality as determined by individual schools. The result is that identical information regarding the facts concerning a particular child is reconstituted anew through distinct professional communications and procedures in each context, as 'the facts' regarding a child's behaviour are utilized for distinct purposes. For example, a crucial distinction between exclusions and special educational needs is that the former focus on what a child has done and can be blamed for, while the latter focus on what a child appears unable to do. Consequently, information regarding a child's conduct in special educational needs is not an end in itself but rather a possible symptom of a condition requiring treatment. Similarly, while the harmful effects of a child's behaviour on other pupils are often the crucial factor in the decision to exclude, it is often irrelevant in the assessment of special educational need. As a result, while an excluded child may be categorized as a child with a special educational need – many are and it is often argued that more should be (Sinclair, 1997; DfEE, 1997) – in the political reconstruction of education, there exists not one 'real' child but two distinct problematized objects of concern constructed and functioning within two separate systems.

Jenks identifies the increased concern about children, their behaviour, standards of education and learning abilities as a reflection not of any dramatic change in children's behaviour but rather as a reflection of complex concerns and deep-rooted anxieties for the future of society. He suggests, and this is of particular relevance in this context, that 'the identification of anomalies is integral to the establishment of social order' (Jenks, 1996, p. 129). Special educational needs and exclusions, and the spiralling increase in the number of children that occupy these 'anomalous' categories consequently reflect the recognition of the interconnection between children's welfare and the well-being of society, as well as the perception that the increasing desire to govern children and childhood is both necessary and legitimate.

These theoretical understandings have crucial implications for practice (Slee, 1997). In particular, they challenge policy-makers to move the focus away from attempts to *solve* the problems of a minority of children, and instead address the complex issues and interests that underlie the construction of the normal child in order to attempt to reconcile anxieties about the future with the possibility of incorporating a plurality of childhoods. An essential precursor for this shift in thinking is the development of reflexive structures that preclude an over-simplification and systematic colonization of the issues and include a genuine form of child responsiveness.

Notes

1 Government in this sense is a reference not to state or government policy but to the Foucauldian notion of governmentality that describes the wide range of disparate practices and techniques by which individuals are regulated and simultaneously regulate themselves (Foucault, 1991; Hunter, 1996; Rose 1996).
2 Education Act 1996 s 527A (as inserted by Education Act 1997 s 9).
3 Education Act 1996 s 156.

4 Education Act s 316.
5 *Gillick v West Norfolk and Wisbech Area Health Authority* [1986] AC 112, [1985] 3 All ER 402, HL.
6 Children Act 1989 s 31.
7 Children Act 1989 s 17.
8 For a discussion of all these factors and others, see Elton (1989).
9 Education Act 1996 s 156.
10 Education Act 1996 Sch 16 para 12A(4) (as inserted by the Education Act 1997 s 7). An example of the appeal committees' wide discretion is provided by *R v Governors of St Gregory's Roman Catholic Aided High School ex p M* [1995] ELR 290. In this case the court held that the permanent exclusion of a pupil for refusing to apologize for swearing in the school playground was neither unreasonable nor disproportionate.
11 Education Act 1996 s 154 (as amended by the Education Act 1997 s 7(3)).
12 Education Act 1996 Sch 16 para 12A(2) (as inserted by the Education Act 1997 s 7).
13 Education Act 1996 s 154 (4),(6),(7) (as substituted by the Education Act 1997 s 2).
14 Education Act 1996 Sch 16 para 12A(1) (as inserted by the Education Act 1997 s 7).
15 *R v Board of Governors of Stoke Newington School, ex p M* [1994] ELR 131.
16 The distinction between education and child care proceedings also demonstrates the limitations placed on the courts by the fact that in education legislation there is no equivalent to the 1989 Children Act's principal and primary provision that the welfare of the child must be the court's paramount consideration: Freeman (1996).
17 Individuals with Disability Education Act 1975/US.
18 Education Act 1996 Sch 16 para 17.
19 Hansard 10/2/97, vol. 578, no. 53, col. 45, HL. See, in particular, the comments of Baronesses Ramsey and Warnock.
20 Education Act 1996 s 411A (as inserted by the Education Act 1997 s 11).
21 Hansard 10/2/97, vol. 578, no. 53, col. 45, HL. See, in particular, the comments of Baronesses Ramsey and Warnock.
22 Education Act 1996 s 316.

Bibliography

Abel, G.G., Becker, J.V. and Cunningham-Rathner, J. (1984) 'Complications, consent and cognitions in sex between children and adults', *International Journal of Law and Psychiatry* 7, 89–103.

Abney, V. and Gunn, D. (1993) 'A rationale for cultural competency', *The APSAC Advisor* 6, 3, 19–22.

Abram, J. (1996) *The Language of Winnicott*, London: Karnac.

Abrams, N. (1979) 'Problems in defining child abuse and neglect', in O'Neill, O. and Ruddick, W. (eds) *Having Children: Philosophical and Legal Reflections on Parenthood*, Oxford: OUP, 156–63.

Aldridge, T. (1994) 'Opinion: repent at pleasure', *Solicitors Journal* 138, 838, 19 August.

Allen, H. (1988) 'One law for all reasonable persons', *International Journal of the Sociology of Law* 16, 4, 149ff.

Archard, D. (1993) *Children, Rights and Childhood*, London: Routledge.

Arey, D. (1995) 'Gay males and sexual child abuse', in Aronson Fontes, L. (ed.) *Sexual Abuse in Nine North American Cultures: Treatment and Prevention*, Thousand Oaks CA: Sage, 200–36.

Ariès, P. (1962) *Centuries of Childhood*, trans. from the French by Robert Baldick, London: Jonathan Cape.

Ashe, M. (1995) 'Postmodernism, legal ethics, and representation of "bad mothers"', in Fineman, M. and Karpin, I. (eds) *Mothers In Law*, New York: Columbia University Press.

Audit Commission (1992) *Getting in on the Act – Provision for Pupils with Special Educational Needs: The National Picture*, London: HMSO.

—— (1996) *Misspent Youth: Young People and Crime*, London: HMSO.

Australian Law Reform Commission (ALRC) *Child Welfare*, Report no. 18, Canberra: Australian Government Printing Service.

Bainham, A. (1988) *Children, Parents and the State*, London: Sweet and Maxwell.

—— (1996) 'Sex education: a family lawyer's perspective', in Harris, N. (ed.) *Children, Sex Education and the Law*, London: National Children's Bureau.

Banks, R. (1997) *The Sweet Hereafter*, London: Vintage.

Bargen, J. (1995) 'A critical view of conferencing', *Australian and New Zealand Journal of Criminology* 25, 100–13.

Bar-On, A. (1997) 'Criminalising survival: images and reality of street children', *Journal of Social Policy* 26, 63.

Baron, S., and Hartnagel, T. (1996) ' "Lock 'em up": attitudes towards punishing juvenile offenders', *Canadian Journal of Criminology* 38, 191–212.

Barron, A. (1996) 'The governance of schooling: genealogies of control and empowerment in the reform of public education', *Studies in Law, Politics and Society* 15, 167–204.

Bart, D. (1984) 'The differential diagnosis of special education: managing social pathology as individual disability', in Barton, L. and Tomlinson S. (eds) *Special Education and Social Interests*, Beckenham: Croom Helm.

Barton, L. and Oliver, M. (1997) 'Special needs: personal trouble or public issue?', in Cosin, B. and Hales, M. (eds) *Families, Education and Social Differences*, London: Routledge.

Barton, L. and Tomlinson, S. (1984) 'The politics of integration in England', in Barton, L and Tomlinson, S. (eds) *Special Education and Social Interests*, Beckenham: Croom Helm.

Bash, L. and Coulby, D. (eds) (1989) *The Education Reform Act: Competition and Control*, London: Cassell.

Bass, E. and Davis, L. (1988) *The Courage to Heal: A Guide for Women Survivors of Child Sexual Abuse*, New York: Harper and Row.

Bauman, Z. (1995) *Life in Fragments*, Oxford: Blackwell.

Becker, H. (1963) *Outsiders*, New York: Free Press of Glencoe.

Behlmer, G.K. (1982) *Child Abuse and Moral Reform in England, 1870–1908*, Stanford, CA: Stanford University Press.

Bell, V. (1993) *Interrogating Incest: Feminism, Foucault and the Law*, London: Routledge.

Bender, L. (1988) 'A lawyer's primer on feminist theory and tort', *Journal of Legal Education* 38, 3.

Berlin, I. (1969) *Four Essays on Liberty*, London: OUP.

Berridge, D. and Brodie, I. (1997) 'An "exclusive" education', *Community Care*, 30 January–5 February, 4.

Bion, W.R. (1962) *Attacks on Linking in Second Thoughts*, New York: Aronson.

Bond, A. (1996) 'Working for the family? Child employment legislation and the public/private divide', *Journal of Social Welfare and Family Law* 18, 3, 291.

Booth, W. (1890) *In Darkest England and the Way Out*, first edition, London: International Headquarters of the Salvation Army.

Bowlby, J.A. (1988) *Secure Base*, London: Routledge.

Boyd, S. (1990) 'Potentialities and perils of the primary caregiver presumption', *Canadian Family Law Quarterly* 7, 1, 1ff.

Boyden, J. (1990) 'Childhood and the policy makers: a comparative perspective on the globalization of childhood', in James, A. and Prout, A. (eds)

Constructing and Reconstructing Childhood: Contemporary Issues in the Sociological Study of Childhood, London: Falmer Press.

Bremner, J. and Hillin, A. (1994) *Sexuality, Young People & Care*, Lyme Regis: Russell House.

Brereton, A. (1997) 'Teaching the unteachable', *Education, Public Law and the Individual* 1, 8.

Britton, R. (1995) 'Psychic reality and unconscious belief', *International Journal of Psycho-Analysis* 76, 19–23.

Brodie, I. (1995) 'Exclusion from school', *Highlight* no. 136, London: National Children's Bureau/Barnardos.

Brongersma, E. (1978) 'From the morality of oppression to creative freedom', *Civis Mundi* 17, 108–15.

Cairns, J. (ed.) (1965) *The Nineteenth Century 1815–1914*, New York: The Free Press.

Calderone, M.S. and Ramey, J.W. (1982) *Talking with Your Child About Sex*, New York: Ballantine.

Califia, P. (1981) 'Man/boy love and the lesbian/gay movement', *The Age Taboo: Gay Male Sexuality, Power and Consent*, London: Gay Men's Press, 133–46.

Campbell, T. (1992) 'The rights of the minor: as person, as child, as future adult', *International Journal of Law and the Family* 6, 1–23.

Cannan, C. (1992) *Changing Families, Changing Welfare*, Hemel Hempstead: Harvester Wheatsheaf.

Cantor, N. (1996) *The Sacred Chain: A History of the Jews*, London: Fontana Press.

Carney, T. (1985) 'The interface between juvenile corrections and child welfare: philosophy pragmatism or professionalisation?', in Borowski, A. and Murray, J. (eds) *Juvenile Delinquency in Australia*, Melbourne: Methuen, 202–220.

—— (1991a) 'Social security: dialogue or closure?', in Alston, P. and Brennan, G. (eds) *The UN Children's Convention and Australia*, Canberra: HREOC, ANU Centre for International and Public Law, ACOSS, 53–61.

—— (1991b) *Law at the Margins: Towards Social Participation*, Melbourne: OUP, 1–199.

—— (1993) 'Special needs children and human rights: relational change under the rights banner?', *Australian Disability Review* 3, 6–21.

—— (1994) 'Client rights and system integrity in the relational state', in Disney, J. and Briggs, L. (eds) *Social Security Policy: Issues and Options*, Canberra: AGPS, 191–208.

—— (1996) 'Welfare appeals and the ARC report: to ssat or not to ssat; is that the question?', *Australian Journal of Administrative Law* 4, 25–36.

—— (1998 in press) 'Merits review of "contractual" social security payments', *Journal of Social Security Law*, forthcoming.

Carney, T. and Tait, D. (1997) *The Adult Guardianship Experiment: Tribunals and Popular Justice*, Sydney: Federation Press.

Carson, W. (1974) 'Symbolic and instrumental dimensions of early factory legislation', in Hood, R. (ed.) *Crime, Criminology and Public Policy*, London: Heinemann.

—— (1980) 'The institutionalisation of ambiguity: early British factory acts', in Geis, G. and Stotland, E. *White Collar Crime: Theory and Research*, London: Sage.

Carvel, J. (1997) 'Exams that create an underclass', *The Guardian*, 21 August.

Chaillou, P. (1989) *Mon Juge*, Paris: Le Pré aux Clercs.

Cheetham, J., James, W., Loney, M., Mayor, B. and Prescott, W. (eds) (1981) *Social & Community Work in a Multi-racial Society*, London: Harper and Row.

Children's Legal Centre (1996) *Banished to the Exclusion Zone*, London: Children's Legal Centre.

Childright (1996) 'School exclusions', *Childright*, no. 132, 6.

Chodorow, N. (1978) *The Reproduction of Mothering*, Berkeley CA and London: The University of California Press.

Clarke, J. and Newman, J. (1993) 'Managing to survive: dilemmas of changing organisational forms in the public sector', in Deakin, N. and Page, R. (eds) *The Costs of Welfare*, Aldershot: Avebury, 46–63.

Coady, C. (1992) 'Theory, rights and children: a comment on O'Neill and Campbell', *International Journal of Law and the Family* 6, 43–51.

Cohen, C. and Miljeteig-Olssen, P. (1991) 'Status report: United Nations Convention on the Rights of the Child', *Journal of Human Rights* 8, 367–82.

Cohen, P. (1992) ' "It's racism what dunnit": hidden narrative in theories of racism', in Rattansi, A. and Donald, J. *'Race' Culture and Difference*, London: Open University and Sage, 62–103.

Cohen, S. (1972) *Folk Devils and Moral Panics*, London: MacGibbon and Kee.

Cooper, A., Hetherington, R., Pitts, J., Baistow, K. and Spriggs, A. (1995) *Positive Child Protection: A View from Abroad*, Lyme Regis: Russell House.

Cooper, D.M. (1993) *Child Abuse Revisited: Children, Society and Social Work*, Buckingham: Open University Press.

Cox, R. (1996) *Shaping Childhood*, London: Routledge.

Cranston, M. (1953) *Freedom: A New Analysis*, London: Longman.

Cunningham, H. (1995) *Children and Childhood in Western Society since 1500*, London: Longman.

Curt, B. (1994) *Textuality and Tectonics: Troubling Social and Psychological Science*, Buckingham: Open University Press.

Dahrendorf, R. (1994) 'The changing quality of citizenship', in Van Steenbergen, B. (ed.) *The Condition of Citizenship*, London: Sage, 10–19.

Davidson, A. (1997) *From Subject to Citizen: Australian Citizenship in the Twentieth Century*, Cambridge: CUP.

Department for Education and Employment (DfEE) (1994a) *Code of Practice on the Identification and Assessment of Children with Special Educational Needs*, London: DfEE.

—— (1994b) *Pupil Behaviour and Discipline*, Circular no. 8/94, London: DfEE.

—— (1994c) *The Education of Children with Emotional and Behavioural Difficulties*, Circular no. 9/94 (DH LAC (94) 9), London: DfEE.

—— (1994d) *Exclusions from School*, Circular no. 10/94, London: DfEE.

—— (1997) *Excellence in Schools*, London: DfEE.

Department of Health and Social Services (1991a) *Working Together:a Guide to Interagency Co-operation for the Protection of Children from Abuse*, London: HMSO.

—— (1991b) *Patient's Charter*, London: HMSO.

Department of Health Social Services Inspectorate (DHSSI) and Office for Standards in Education (OFSTED) (1995) *The Education of Children who are Looked After by Local Authorities*, London: Department of Health.

Diamantides, M. (1995) 'Ethics in law. Death marks on a still-life. A vision of judgement as vegetating', *Law and Critique* 5, 209–28.

Diduck, A. (1999) 'Conceiving the bad mother: the focus should be on the child to be born', *University of British Columbia Law Review* 32 (forthcoming).

Dingwall, R. and Eekelaar, J. (1984) 'Rethinking child protection', in Freeman, M. (ed.) *The State, the Law and the Family: Critical Perspectives*, London: Tavistock Publications, 93–114.

Dingwall, R., Eekelaar, J. and Murray, T. (1984) 'Childhood as a social problem: a survey of the history of legal regulation', *Journal of Law and Society* 11, 207–32.

—— (1995) *The Protection of Children*, second edition, Aldershot: Avebury.

Dominelli, L. (1988) *Anti-Racist Social Work*, London: Macmillan.

—— (1989) 'Betrayal of trust: a feminist analysis of power relationships in incest abuse and its relevance to social work practice', *British Journal of Social Work* 19, 295–332.

Donzelot, J. (1980) *The Policing of Families*, London: Hutchinson.

Dorkenoo, E. and Elworthy, S. (1992) *Female Genital Mutilation: Proposals for Change*, London: Minority Rights Group International.

Dresser, M. (1997) 'The painful rite: Jewish circumcision in English thought 1753–1945', *The Jewish Quarterly*, Summer, 15–17.

Dutt, R. and Phillips, M. (1996) 'Race, culture and the prevention of child abuse', in *National Commission of Inquiry into the Prevention of Child Abuse: Childhood Matters: vol. 2: Background Papers*, London: The Stationery Office, 148–201.

Dworkin, G. (1974) 'Non-neutral principles', *The Journal of Philosophy* 71, 491–506.

Eekelaar, J. (1986) 'The emergence of children's rights', *Oxford Journal of Legal Studies*, 6, 161–82.

—— (1992) 'The importance of thinking that children have rights', in Alston, P., Parker, S. and Seymour. J. (eds) *Children, Rights and the Law*, Oxford: Clarendon Press.

Eekelaar, J., Dingwall, R. and Murray, T. (1982) 'Victims or threats? Children in care proceedings', *Journal of Social Welfare Law*, 68–82.

Elton, Lord (1989) *Discipline in Schools* (Report of the Committee of Inquiry chaired by Lord Elton), London: HMSO.

Escott, T. (1881) *England: Its People, Polity and Pursuits*, London: Cassell.

Fairbairn, W.R.D. (1954) *Psychoanalytic Studies of the Personality*, London: Routledge.

Ferry, J-M. (1994) 'Approaches to liberty: outline for a "methodological communitarianism"', *Ratio Juris* 7, 291–307.

Finch, J. (1984) *Education as Social Policy*, London: Longman.

Fineman, M. (1995) 'Preface', in Fineman, M. and Karpin, I. (eds) *Mothers In Law*, New York: Columbia University Press.

Finkelhor, D. and Korbin, J. (1988) 'Child abuse as an international issue', *Child Abuse and Neglect* 12, 3–23.

Finlayson, G. (1994) *Citizen, State and Social Welfare in Britain, 1830–1990*, Oxford: Clarendon Press.

Fitzpatrick, P. (1998) 'Missing possibility: socialisation, culture and consciousness', presentation to Law and Society Association Summer Institute in *Crossing Boundaries: Traditions and Transformations in Law and Society Research*, Evanston, IL: Northwestern University Press.

Foucault, M. (1973) *The Birth of the Clinic: An Archaeology of Medical Perception*, New York: Vintage.

—— (1990) *History of Sexuality*, vol. I, Harmondsworth: Penguin.

—— (1991) 'Governmentality', in Burchell, G., Gordon, C. and Miller, P. (eds) *The Foucault Effect, Studies in Governmentality*, London: Harvester Wheatsheaf.

Fraser, N. and Gordon, L. (1994) 'Civil citizenship against social citizenship? On the ideology of contract-versus-charity', in Van Steenbergen, B. (ed.) *The Condition of Citizenship*, London: Sage, 90–107.

Freeman, M. (1983) *The Rights and Wrongs of Children*, London: Frances Pinter.

—— (1992) 'Taking children's rights more seriously', in Alston, P., Parker, S. and Seymour, J. (eds) *Children, Rights and the Law*, Oxford: Clarendon Press.

—— (1995) 'The morality of cultural pluralism', *The International Journal of Children's Rights* 3, 1–17.

—— (1996) 'The convention: an English perspective', in Freeman, M. (ed.) *Children's Rights: A Comparative Perspective*, Aldershot: Dartmouth.

Freud, S. (1923) *The Ego and the Id*, London, Standard Edition, xix, 3–66.

—— ([1933] 1964) 'Introductory lecture 32: anxiety and its instinctual life', in *Collected Works*, standard edition, vol. XXII, London: Hogarth Press and Institute of Psychoanalysis.

Frosh, S. (1997) *For and Against Psychoanalysis*, London: Routledge.

Frug, M.J. (1992) *Postmodern Legal Feminism*, London: Routledge.

Furniss, T (1991) *The Multi-Professional Handbook of Child Sexual Abuse*, London: Routledge.

Galloway, D., Armstrong, D. and Tomlinson, S. (1994) *The Assessment of Special Educational Needs – Whose Problem?*, London: Longman.

Gamble, H. (1985) 'The status offender', in Borowski, A. and Murray, J. (eds) *Juvenile Delinquency in Australia*, Melbourne: Methuen, 95–111.

Garapon, A. (1989) 'Modèle garantiste et modèle paternaliste dans les systèmes de justice des mineurs', *Actes* 66, 19–24.

Garbarino, J., Guttman, E. and Shelley, J. (1986) *The Psychologically Battered Child*, San Francisco: Jossey-Bass.

Garlock, P. (1979) 'Wayward children and the law 1820–1900: the genesis of the status offence jurisdiction of the juvenile court', *Georgia Law Review* 13, 341–447.

Gelles, R.J. (1975) 'The social construction of child abuse', *American Journal of Orthopsychiatry*, 45, 363–71.

Gellner, E. (1992) *Postmodernism, Reason and Religion*, London and New York: Routledge.

Gerrard, N. (1997) 'Little girls lost', *The Observer*, Review section, 31 August.

Gil, D. (1975) 'Unravelling child abuse', *American Journal of Orthopsychiatry* 45, 346–56.

Gilligan, C. (1982) *In a Different Voice*, Cambridge MA: Harvard University Press.

Gilroy, P. (1987) *There Ain't no Black in the Union Jack*, London: Routledge.

Goodin, R. and Le Grande, J. (1987) *Not Only the Poor*, London: Allen and Unwin.

Gordon, L. (1988) *Heroes of Their Own Lives*, New York: Viking Penguin.

Gough, D. (1996) 'Defining the problem', *Child Abuse and Neglect* 20, 993–1002.

Gough, D. and Murray, K. (1996) 'The research literature on the prevention of child abuse', in *Childhood Matters, Report of the National Commission of Inquiry into the Prevention of Child Abuse: vol. 2: Background Papers*, London: The Stationery Office, 203ff.

Gough, J. (1981) 'Childhood, sexuality and pedophilia', in *The Age Taboo: Gay Male Sexuality, Power and Consent*, London: Gay Men's Press, 65–71.

Govier, T. (1992) *A Practical Study of Argument*, third edition, Belmont CA: Wadsworth Publishing Company.

Gray, J. (1996), *After Social Democracy*, London: Demos.

Gusfield, J. (1963) *Symbolic Crusade*, Urbana: University of Illinois Press.

Habermas, J. (1984) *The Theory of Communicative Action*, vol. 1, Boston: Beacon Press.

—— (1987) *The Theory of Communicative Action*, vol. 2, Cambridge: CUP.

Hacking, I. (1988) 'The sociology of knowledge about child abuse', *Noûs* 22, 53–63.

—— (1991) 'The making and molding of child abuse', *Critical Inquiry* 17, 253–88.

Hand, S. (ed.) (1989) *The Levinas Reader*, Oxford: Blackwell.

Handler, J. (1988) 'Dependent people, the state, and the modern/postmodern search for the dialogic community', *UCLA Law Review* 35, 999–1113.

Harland, J. and Kinder, K. (1995) 'Buzzes and barriers: young people's attitudes to participation in the arts', *Children and Society* 9, 4, 15–31.

Harris, D. (1987) *Justifying State Welfare: The New Right Versus the Old Left*, Oxford: Basil Blackwell.

Harris, N. (1993a) *Law and Education: Regulation, Consumerism and the Education System*, London: Sweet and Maxwell.

—— (1993b) 'Social citizenship and young people in Europe', in Jackson, B. and McGoldrick, D. (eds) *Legal Visions of the New Europe*, London: Graham and Trotman/Martinus Nijhoff, 185–224.

—— (1997a) *Special Educational Needs and Access to Justice*, Bristol: Jordans.

—— (1997b) 'Education and judicial review – an overview', *Education, Public Law and the Individual* 5, 24–7.

Harris, R. and Parsons, C. (1998) *Excluded Children*, London: Routledge.

Harrison, B. (1991) 'Drug addiction in pregnancy: the interface of science, emotion and social policy', *Journal of Substance Abuse Treatment*, 8, 261.

Hart, H.L.A. (1961) *The Concept of Law*, Oxford: Clarendon Press.

Hay, C. (1995) 'Mobilization through interpellation: James Bulger, juvenile crime and the construction of moral panic', *Social and Legal Studies* 4, 197–223.

Hayden, C. (1994) 'Primary age children excluded from school: a multi-agency focus for concern', *Children and Society* 8, 3, 257–73.

Hendrick, H. (1990) 'Constructions and reconstructions of childhood: an interpretive survey, 1800 to the present', in James, A. and Prout, A. (eds) *Constructing and Reconstructing Childhood: Contemporary Issues in the Sociological Study of Childhood*, London: Falmer Press.

—— (1994) *Child Welfare, England 1872–1989*, London: Routledge.

Hetherington, R., Cooper, A., Smith, P. and Wilford, G. (1997), *Protecting Children: Messages from Europe*, Lyme Regis: Russell House.

Himmelfarb, G. (1995) *The De-moralisation of Society: From Victorian Virtues to Modern Values*, London: IEA Health and Welfare Unit.

Hindle, D. (1994) 'Learning to think in a "war zone"', *Journal of Child Psychotherapy* 20, 3 , 343–57.

Hodgkin, R. (1997) 'The Education Act and excluded children', *Children and Society* 11, 135–7.

Hoffman, L.A. (1996) *Covenant of Blood: Circumcision and Gender in Rabbinic Judaism*, Chicago: University of Chicago Press.

Hollingsworth, E. (1996) 'Mental health services in England: the 1990s', *International Journal of Law and Psychiatry* 19, 309–25.

Horsburgh, M. (1980) 'The apprenticing of dependent children in NSW between 1850–1885', *Journal of Australian Studies* 7, 34–5.

Hoskin, K. (1990) 'Foucault under examination: the crypto-educationalist unmasked', in Ball, S. (ed.) *Foucault and Education: Disciplines and Knowledge*, London: Routledge.

Hunter, I. (1996) 'Assembling the school', in Barry, A., Osborne, T. and Rose, N. (eds) *Foucault and Political Reason*, London: UCL.

Jackson, V. (1996) *Racism and Child Protection: The black Experience of Child Abuse*, London: Cassell.

James, A. and Jenks, C. (1996) 'Public perceptions of childhood criminality', *British Journal of Sociology* 47, 315–31.

James, A. and Prout, A. (1997) 'A new paradigm for the sociology of child-hood', in James and Prout (eds) *Constructing and Reconstructing Childhood: Contemporary Issues in the Sociology of Childhood*, London: Falmer Press.

Jeffs, T. (1995) 'Children's educational rights in a new ERA?', in Franklin, B. (ed.) *The Handbook of Children's Rights: Comparative Policy and Practice*, London: Routledge.

Jenks, C. (1996) *Childhood*, London: Routledge.

Katz, I. (1996a) 'The sociology of children from minority ethnic communities – issues and methods', in Butler, I. and Shaw, I. *A Case of Neglect? Children's Experience and the Sociology of Childhood*, London: Avebury.

—— (1996b) *The Construction of Racial Identity in Children of Mixed Parentage – Mixed Metaphors*, London: Jessica Kingsley.

Keats, D.M. (1997) *Culture and the Child: A Guide for Professionals in Child Care and Development*, Chichester: Wiley.

Kempe, H.C. *et al.* (1962) 'The Battered Child Syndrome', *Journal of the American Medical Association*, 181, 17–24.

Kennedy, R. (1997) *Child Abuse, Psychotherapy and the Law*, London: Free Association Books.

King, M. (1981) 'Welfare and justice', in King, M. (ed.) *Childhood, Welfare and Justice*, London: Batsford Academic, 105–36.

—— (ed.) (1995) *God's Law versus State Law: The Construction of an Islamic Identity in Western Europe*, London: Grey Seal.

—— (1997) *A Better World for Children, Explorations in Morality and Authority*, London: Routledge.

King, M. and Piper, C. (1995) *How the Law Thinks about Children*, second edition, Aldershot: Arena.

King, M. and Schütz, A. (1994) 'The ambitious modesty of Niklas Luhmann', *Journal of Law and Society* 21, 261.

King, M. and Trowell, J. (1992) *Children's Welfare and the Law: The Limits of Legal Intervention*, London: Sage.

Kitson-Clarke, G. (1962) *The Making of Victorian England*, London: Methuen.

Klein, M.([1921] [1928] 1975) *The Development Of A Child* [1921] and *Early Stages of the Oedipal Conflict* [1928], in *Love, Guilt & Reparation*, London: Hogarth Press.

—— ([1935] 1975) *A Contribution to the Psychogenesis of Manic-depressive States*, in *Love, Guilt & Reparation*, London: Hogarth Press.

—— ([1945] 1965) *The Oedipal Complex in the Light of Early Anxieties*, in *Love, Guilt & Reparation*, London: Hogarth Press.

Korbin, J.E. (ed.) (1981) *Child Abuse and Neglect: Cross Cultural Perspectives* Berkeley CA: University of California Press.

—— (1993) 'Cultural diversity and child maltreatment', *The APSAC Advisor* 6, 3, 23–4.

Kosonen, P. (1995) 'European welfare state models: converging trends', *International Journal of Sociology* 25, 25, 81–110.

Kritzman, L.D. (1988) *Michel Foucault: Politics, Philosophy, Culture: Interviews and Other Writings 1977–84*, New York: Routledge.

Kymlicka, W. and Norman, W. (1994) 'Return of the citizen: a survey of recent work on citizenship theory', *Ethics* 104, 352–81.

Kyrle, M. (1932) *The Development of Sexual Impulses*, London: Kegan Paul.

La Prairie, C. (1995) 'Altering course: new directions in criminal justice; sentencing circles and family group conferences', *Australian and New Zealand Journal of Criminology* 25, Spring, 78–99.

Latham, M. (1996) 'Making welfare work', paper delivered to the Centre for Independent Studies, Melbourne University, 31 July.

LeBlanc, L. (1995) *The Convention on the Rights of the Child, United Nations Lawmaking on Human Rights*, Lincoln NE and London: University of Nebraska Press.

Leisink, P. and Coenen, H. (1993) 'Work and citizenship in the New Europe', in Coenen, H. and Leisink, P. (eds) *Work and Citizenship in the New Europe*, Aldershot: Edward Elgar, 1–32.

Levinas, E. (1969) *Totality and Infinity*, trans. by A. Lingis, The Hague: Martinus Nijhoff.

—— (1986) 'The trace of the other', trans. by A. Lingis, in Taylor, M. (ed.) *Deconstruction in Context*, Chicago: University of Chicago Press.

Lewis, J. (1992) 'Women in late nineteenth century social work', in Smart, C. (ed.) *Regulating Womanhood: Historical Essays on Marriage, Motherhood and Sexuality*, London: Routledge.

Lightfoot-Klein, H. (1989) *Prisoners of Ritual: An Odyssey into Female Genital Circumcision in Africa*, Binghampton NY: Harrington Park Press.

Lloyd, G. (1984) *The Man of Reason: 'Male' and 'Female' in Western Philosophy*, London: Methuen.

Lorenz, C. (1997) 'Tough at the top – the problems faced by exceptionally able children', *Education, Public Law and Individuals*, 1, 2.

Luhmann, N. (1986) 'The autopoiesis of social systems', in Geyer, F. and van der Zouwen, J. (eds) *Sociocybernetic Paradoxes: Observation, Control and Evolution of Self-Steering Systems*, London and Beverly Hills: Sage.

—— (1989) *Ecological Communications*, Oxford: Polity.

—— (1993a) 'The code of the moral', *Cardozo Law Review* 14, 995.

—— (1993b) *Risk: A Sociological Theory*, New York: Aldine de Gruyter.

—— (1994) 'Politicians, and the higher amorality of politics', *Theory, Culture and Society* 11, 25.

—— (1995) *Social Systems*, Stanford CA: Stanford University Press.

McDiarmid, C. (1996) 'A feminist perspective on children who kill', *Res Publica* 2, 1, 3ff.

McGillivray, A. (1997) 'Governing childhood', in McGillivray, A. (ed.) *Governing Childhood*, Aldershot: Dartmouth.

McGoldrick, D. (1991) 'The United Nations Convention on the Rights of the Child', *International Journal of Law and the Family* 5, 132–69.

MacIntyre, A. (1981) *After Virtue: A Study in Moral Theory*, London: Duckworth.

Machiavelli, N. (1532) 'The Prince', in Bondanella, P. and Musa, M. (eds) (1979) *The Portable Machiavelli*, Harmondsworth: Penguin.

Mandela, N. (1994) *Long Walk to Freedom: The Autobiography of Nelson Mandela*, Randburg South Africa: Macdonald Purnell.

Marneffe, C. (1992) 'The confidential doctor centre – a new approach to child protection work', *Adoption & Fostering* 16, 4, 23–8.

Marshall, T. (1973) *Sociology at the Crossroads and Other Essays*, London: Heinemann, 67–127.

Marvell, H. (1977) 'Factory regulation: a reinterpretation of early English experience', *Journal of Law and Economics* 20, 379–402.

Metcalf, S. (1994) 'Children who kill', *Australian Journal of Forensic Sciences* 26, 38–42.

Mnookin, R. (1985) 'Divorce bargaining: the limits of private ordering', *Michigan Journal of Law Reform* 18, 1015–35.

Money, J. (1985) *The Destroying Angel*, Buffalo NY: Prometheus Books.

Monk, D. (1997) 'School exclusions and the Education Act 1997', *Education and the Law* 9, 4: 277–290.

—— (1998) 'Sex education and the problematisation of teenage pregnancy: a genealogy of law and governance', *Social and Legal Studies* 7, 2, 241–61.

Monture, P. (1989) 'A vicious circle: child welfare law and the first nations', *Canadian Journal of Women and the Law* 3, 1.

Moon, J. (1993) 'Citizenship and welfare: social democratic and liberal perspectives', in Wilson, W. (ed.) *Sociology and the Public Agenda*, Newbury Park CA: Sage, 97–118.

Morgan, J. (1986) 'Controlling minors' fertility', *Monash University Law Review* 12, 161–97.

Morris, A. and Maxwell, G. (1993) 'Juvenile justice in New Zealand: a new paradigm', *Australian and New Zealand Journal of Criminology* 26, 72–90.

Morrison, B. (1994) 'Children of circumstance', *The New Yorker* 69, 14 February, 48–60.

Mossman, M.J. (1991) 'Feminism and legal method: the difference it makes', in Fineman, M. and Thomadsen, N. (eds) *At the Boundaries of Law: Feminism and Legal Theory*, London: Routedge.

Mowat, C.L. (1961) *The Charity Organisation Society 1869–1913*, London: Methuen.

Murray, J. (1985) 'The development of contemporary juvenile justice and correctional policy', in Borowski, A. and Murray, J. (eds) *Juvenile Delinquency in Australia*, Melbourne: Methuen, 68–89.

Naffine, N. (1990) *Law and the Sexes: Explorations in Feminist Jurisprudence*, Sydney: Allen and Unwin.

—— (1992) 'Children in the children's court: can there be rights without a remedy?', *International Journal of Law and the Family* 6, 76–97.

National Commission of Inquiry into the Prevention of Child Abuse (1996) *Childhood Matters*, vol. 1, London: The Stationery Office.

Nelken, D. (1987) 'The use of "contracts" as a social work technique', *Current Legal Problems* 40, 207–32.

Nelson, S. (1987) *Incest: Fact and Myth*, second edition, Edinburgh: Stramullion.

Norrie, A. (1993) *Crime, Reason and History: A Critical Introduction to Criminal Law*, London: Weidenfeld and Nicolson.

—— (1996) 'The limits of justice: finding fault in the criminal law', *Modern Law Review* 59, 540.

O'Carroll, T. (1980) *Paedophilia: The Radical Case*, London: Peter Own.

O'Connor, I. (1997) 'Models of juvenile justice', in Borowski, A. and O'Connor, I. (eds) *Juvenile Crime, Justice and Corrections*, Sydney: Longman, 229–53.

Odhams (*c.* 1954) *Odhams Encyclopaedia for Children*, Watford: Odhams.

O'Dell, L. (1997) 'Child sexual abuse and the academic construction of symptomatologies', *Feminism and Psychology* 7, 3, 334–9.

O'Donovan, K. (1985) *Sexual Divisions in Law*, London: Weidenfeld and Nicolson.

—— (1993) *Family Law Matters*, London: Pluto Press.

Oldfield, A. (1990) 'Citizenship: an unnatural practice?', *Political Quarterly* 61, 177–87.

Oliver, S. and Austen, L. (1996) *Special Educational Needs and the Law*, Bristol: Jordans.

Olsen, F. (1983) 'The family and the market: a study of ideology and legal reform', *Harvard Law Review* 96, 1560.

O'Neill, O. (1992) 'Children's rights and children's lives', *International Journal of Law and the Family* 6, 24–42.

O'Sullivan, T., Hartley, J., Saunders, D., Montgomery, M. and Fiske, J. (1994) *Key Concepts in Communication and Cultural Studies*, second edition, London: Routledge.

Palmer, S. (1996). 'What has happened to children's rights in the criminal justice system?', *Cambridge Law Journal* 55, 406–9.

Parker, G. (1976) 'The juvenile court movement', *University of Toronto Law Journal* 26, 140–72.

Parkinson, P. (1997) *Child Sexual Abuse and the Churches*, London: Hodder and Stoughton.

Parsons, C. (1996) 'Permanent exclusions from schools in England in the 1990s: trends, causes and responses', *Children and Society* 10, 177–86.

Parton, N. (1985) *The Politics of Child Abuse*, London: Macmillan.

Parton, N., Thorpe, D. and Wattam, C. (1997) *Child Protection: Risk and the Moral Order*, Basingstoke: Macmillan.

Pfohl, S.J. (1977) 'The "discovery" of child abuse', *Social Problems* 24, 310–23.

Pinchbeck, I. and Hewitt, M. (1969) *Children in English Society: vol 1: From Tudor Times to the 18th Century*, London: Routledge and Kegan Paul.

—— (1973) *Children in English Society: vol. 2: From the 18th Century to the Children Act*, London: Routledge and Kegan Paul.

Pixley, J. (1993) *Citizenship and Employment: Investigating Post-Industrial Options*, Hong Kong: CUP.

Platt, A. (1969) *The Child Savers: The Invention of Delinquency*, Chicago: University of Chicago Press.

—— (1977) *The Child Savers: The Invention of Delinquency*, second edition, Chicago: University of Chicago Press.

Pollock, L. (1983) *Forgotten Children: Parent-child relations from 1500 to 1900*, Cambridge: CUP.

Prager, J. (1992) 'Contracting-out: theory and policy', *New York University Journal of International Law and Politics* 25, 73–111.

Ramsland, J. (1986) *Children of the Backlanes: Destitute and Neglected Children in Colonial New South Wales*, Kensington Australia: University of NSW Press.

Rattansi, A. (1992) 'Changing the subject? Racism, culture and education', in Rattansi, A. and Donald, J. (eds) *'Race' Culture and Difference*, London: Open University and Sage, 11–48.

Rees, A. (1995) 'The promise of social citizenship', *Policy and Politics* 23, 313–25.

Reich, C. (1964) 'The new property', *Yale Law Journal* 73, 733–87.

Richards, N. (1997) 'Criminal children', *Law and Philosophy* 16, 63–89.

Riddell, S. and Brown, S. (eds) (1994) *Special Educational Needs Policy in the 1990s*, London: Routledge.

Robinson, K. (1995) 'Children, society and the arts', *Children and Society* 9, 4, 5–14.

Robinson, R. (1965) *Definition*, Oxford: OUP.

Rodham, H. (1973) 'Children under the law', *Harvard Educational Review* 43, 487–514.

Rose, N. (1989) *Governing the Soul – The Shaping of the Private Self*, London: Routledge.

—— (1996) 'The death of the social? Refiguring the territory of government', *Economy and Society* 25, 3, 327–56.

Rose, W. (1994) Paper presented to the 'Working for Children' Conference, Cumberland Lodge, Windsor.

Rothman, B. (1989) *Recreating Motherhood: Ideology and Technology in Patriarchal Society*, New York: WW Norton.

Royal College of Nursing (1994) *Female Genital Mutilation: The Unspoken Issue*, London Royal College of Nursing.

Russell, P. (1990) 'The Education Reform Act – the implications for special educational needs', in Flude, M. and Russell, P. (eds) *The Education Reform Act, 1988. Its Origins and Implications*, London: Falmer Press.

Sahgal, G. and Yuval-Davis, N. (eds) (1992) *Refusing Holy Orders*, London: Virago.

Sampford, C. (1986) 'The dimensions of liberty and their judicial protection', *Law in Context* 4, 29–51.

Sandow, S. (1990) 'The pre-school years: early intervention and prevention', in Evans, P. and Varma, V. (eds) *Special Education: Past, Present and Future*, London: Falmer Press.

Sarat, A. (1997) 'Vengeance, victims and the identities of law', *Social and Legal Studies* 6, 2, 163–89.

Scharff, D. (1966) *Object Relations Theory & Practice*, New York: Aronson.

Schechter, M. and Roberge, L. (1976) 'Sexual exploitation', in Helfer, R. and Kempe, C. (eds) *Child Abuse and Neglect: The Family and Community*, Cambridge MA.: Ballinger Publishing, 127–42.

Schonefeld, V. (1995) *It's a Boy!*, video, Channel 4 television.

Schools Curriculum and Assessment Authority (SCAA) (1995) *Spiritual and Moral Development*, Discussion Paper no. 3.

—— (1996) *Education for Adult Life: The Spiritual and Moral Development of Young People*, Discussion Paper no. 6.

Semmell, B. (1960) *Imperialism and Social Reform 1895–1914*, London: Allen and Unwin.

Seymour, J. (1985) 'Children's courts in Australia', in Borowski, A. and Murray, J. (eds) *Juvenile Delinquency in Australia*, Melbourne: Methuen, 186–201.

—— (1988) *Dealing with Young Offenders*, Sydney: Law Book Company.

Sherman, A. (1997) 'Five-year-olds' perception of why we go to school', *Children and Society* 11, 2, 117–27.

Silver, R. (1997) 'Attention deficit hyperactivity disorder', *Family Law*, August, 547–50.

Simey, M. (1951) *Charitable Effort in Liverpool in the 19th Century*, Liverpool: Liverpool University Press.

Simon, W. (1983) 'Legality, bureaucracy, and class in the welfare system', *Yale Law Journal* 92, 1198–269.

—— (1986) 'Rights and redistribution in the welfare system', *Stanford Law Review* 38, 1431–516.

Sinclair, R. (1997) 'School exclusions: working together', *Community Care* 30 January–5 February, 1.

Singer, J. (1992) 'The privatization of family law', *Wisconsin Law Review* v–vi, 1443–57.

Slee, Roger (1995) *Changing Theories and Practices of Discipline*, London: Falmer Press.

—— (1997) 'Imported or important theory? Sociological interrogations of disablement and special education', *British Journal of Sociology of Education* 18, 3, 407–19.

Smart, C. (1991) 'The legal and moral ordering of child custody', *Journal of Law and Society* 18, 485.

Spargo, J. [1906] (1969) *The Bitter Cry of the Children*, New York: Johnson Reprint Corporation.

Spock, B. (1963) *Baby and Child Care*, Montreal: Pocket Books.

Stainton Rogers, R. and Stainton Rogers, W. (1992) *Stories of Childhood: Shifting Agendas of Child Concern*, Hemel Hempstead: Harvester Wheatsheaf.

Stainton Rogers, W. and Stainton Rogers, R. (1996) 'Children + adults + sex = ?', paper presented at the symposium on Child Sexual Abuse, Department of Social Anthropology, University of Edinburgh, May.

Stevenson, C.L. 'Persuasive definitions', *Mind* 47 (July 1938), 331–50.

Stewart, A. (1995) 'Two conceptions of citizenship', *British Journal of Sociology* 46, 63–78.

Sullivan, T. (1992) *Sexual Abuse and the Rights of Children: Reforming Canadian Law*, Toronto: University of Toronto Press.

Sumner, L.W. (1987) *The Moral Foundation of Rights*, Oxford: Clarendon Press.

Sutton, A. (1981) 'The social role of educational psychology in the definition of educational subnormality', in Barton, L. and Tomlinson, S. (eds) *Special Education: Policy, Practices and Social Issues*, London: Harper and Row.

Teubner, G. (1993) *Law as an Autopoietic System*, Oxford: Blackwell.

Theweleit, K. (1977) *Male Fantasies*, Cambridge: Polity.

Thomas, G. and Davis, P. (1997) 'Special needs: objective reality or personal construction? Judging reading difficulty after the Code of Practice', *Educational Research* 39, 3, 263–71.

Thompson, B. (1994) *Soft Core: Moral Crusades against Pornography in Britain and America*, London: Cassell.

Thorpe, D. and Jackson, M. (1997) 'Child protection services and parental reactions to children's behaviour', *Child and Family Social Work* 2, 81–9.

Tomlinson, S. (1981) *Educational Subnormality*, London: Routledge and Kegan Paul.

Tosh, J. (1995) *The Pursuit of History*, second edition, London: Longman.

Tyler, D. (1997) 'At risk of maladjustment: the problem of child mental health', in Peterson, A. and Bunton, R. (eds) *Foucault: Health and Medicine*, London: Routledge.

Van Gunsteren, H. (1994) 'Four conceptions of citizenship', in Van Steenbergen, B. (ed.) *The Condition of Citizenship*, London: Sage, 36–48.

Visser, J. (1993) 'A broad, balanced, relevant and differentiated curriculum', in Visser, J. and Upton, G. (eds) *Special Education in Britain after Warnock*, London: David Fulton.

Walby, S. (1995) 'Gender, work and post-Fordism: the EC context', *International Journal of Sociology* 25, 67–82.

Walgrave, L. (1996) 'Restorative juvenile justice', in Asquith, A. (ed.) *Children and Young People in Conflict with the Law*, London: Jessica Kingsley, 169–99.

Walling, W. H. (1909) *Sexology*, Philadelphia: Puritan.

Walzer, M. (1983) *Spheres of Justice*, New York: Basic Books.

Ward, J. (1970) *The Factory System*, vol. 2, Newton Abbot: David and Charles.

Warnock, M. (1978) *Special Educational Needs: Report of the Committee of Enquiry into the Education of Handicapped Children and Young People*, London: HMSO.

Weatherley, R. (1994) 'From entitlement to contract: reshaping the welfare state in Australia', *Journal of Sociology and Social Welfare* 21, 153–73.

Webb, B. (1926) *My Apprenticeship*, London: Longman.

Wedell, K. (1990) 'Children with special educational needs: past, present and future', in Evans, P. and Varma, V. (eds) *Special Education: Past, Present and Future*, London: Falmer Press.

Weinberg, J. (1995) 'Older mothers and adult children: toward an alternative construction of care', in Fineman, M. and Karpin, I. (eds) *Mothers In Law*, New York: Columbia University Press.

Weintraub, J. (1990) 'The theory and politics of the public/private distinction', unpublished paper presented to the American Political Science Association.

Weisz, V. (1995) *Children and Adolescents in Need: A Legal Primer for the Helping Professional*, London: Sage.

West, D.J. (1967) *The Young Offenders*, Harmondsworth: Penguin.

Whelan, R. (1996) *The Corrosion of Charity: From Moral Renewal to Contract Culture*, London: IEA Health and Welfare Unit.

White, R., Underwood, R. and Omelczuk, S. (1991) 'Victims of violence: the view from the youth services', *Australian and New Zealand Journal of Criminology* 24, 25–39.

Wilkinson, H. and Mulgan, G. (1995) *Freedom's Children: Work, Relationships and Politics for 18–34 Year Olds in Britain Today*, London: Demos.

Wilson, W. (1994) 'Citizenship and the inner-city ghetto poor', in Van Steenbergen, B. (ed.) *The Condition of Citizenship*, London: Sage, 49–65.

Winnicott, D.W. ([1935] 1958) *The Manic Defence*, in *Collected Papers*, London: Tavistock Publications.

—— ([1945] 1958) *Primitive Emotional Development*, in *Collected Papers*, London: Tavistock Publications.

—— ([1962] 1976) 'Ego integration in child development', in *Maturational Processes and the Facilitating Environment*, London: Hogarth Press.

Woodhouse, B. (1993) 'Children's rights: The destruction and promise of family', *Brigham Young University Law Review*, no volume, 497–515.

Wyn, J. and White, R. (1997) *Rethinking Youth*, London: Sage.

Yeatman, A. (1995) 'Interpreting contemporary contractualism', in Boston, J. (ed.) *The State Under Contract*, Wellington: Bridget Williams, 124–39.

Yngvesson, B. (1997) 'Negotiating motherhood: identity and difference in "open" adoptions', *Law and Society Review* 31, 33.

Young, A. (1996) *Imagining Crime: Textual Outlaws and Criminal Conversations*, London: Sage.

Žižek, S. (1989) *The Sublime Object of Ideology*, London: Verso.

—— (1991) *Looking Awry*, Cambridge MA: MIT Press.

Author index

Subject index

aboriginal children 25, 125
abuse *see* child abuse, sexual abuse
adolescents, dilemmas for psychoanalysts 150–1
adults: moral agendas and the child 15, 16; reformulation of boundary between adulthood and childhood 121–33; *see also* parents
agency 132–3; human action and child abuse 76, 78, 83
anorexia 115, 150–1
anti-fundamentalism 209–10
anti-humanism 203
anti-racism 94, 97–8, 208
anti-Semitism 98–9
anti-therapeutic therapy 145
assessment 222
attachment theory 149, 150
attention deficit disorder (ADD) 223
Australia 25, 54, 125, 193
authority: absolute and fundamentalism 201–2; child welfare professionals and 156–8
autopoietic theory 6–7, 226–7

behavioural difficulties 31–2, 212–29
Belgium 164–7, 169
Bulger, James 56, 60, 126–7

Calvin Klein advertising campaign 194
campaigns, moral *see* moral campaigns
Canada 25, 54, 125, 192–3, 195

capacity rights 68
care proceedings under the Children Act 1989 217; *see also* child protection, systems and justice
Carpenter, Mary 33, 54
child abuse 19–21, 74–89; 'battered babies' 183; collective 78–9, 83; community norm for 86; construction and energization of 183–4; defining harms to children 75–7; discursive production 184–8; new forms of 79; non-contentiousness 77–9; orthodox and persuasive definitions 79–81; physical 80, 93, 103; problems of fixing meanings 81–7; reasons for defining 74–5; sexual abuse 80, 181–2; therapists and confidentiality 146–7; *see also* child protection
child autonomy 123; dependence, agency and 132–3; Gillick case and 116, 118–19; parenting and 23–4, 110–11; *see also* rights
child care proceedings 217
child development: cognitive 191, 221; scientific theories of 222
child labour 36–9, 54, 128
child maturity 115
child protection: and circumcision 91, 95–6; protectionist discourse 181–4, 192–3, 195; psychoanalytic practice and

142–5; systems and justice 26–8, 154–78
child saving policies 57–9
child sexuality *see* sexuality
child welfare 18–19, 53–73;
    changing conceptions of the
    welfare state 59–67; changing
    moral pictures of childhood 54–7;
    child saving policies 57–9;
    citizenship 59–61;
    communitarianism 66–7;
    contractualism 61–4;
    postmodernism 64–6;
    professionals and authority 156–8
child's capacity to understand 115
child's needs 58; basic 85–6; special
    educational needs 31–2, 212–13,
    220–5, 225–8
child's vulnerability 36, 108
childhood 53; changing moral
    pictures of 54–7; crisis of 25,
    127–32; fundamentalism and
    children 205–7; images of *see*
    images of children; reformulation
    of boundaries between adulthood
    and 121–33; visibility of the
    Victorian child 35–9
childminders 42–3
Children Act 1989 85, 142, 168,
    192; child care proceedings 217
children's courts 54–5, 57–8, 160–1
Children's Judge 160, 164, 169
children's rights *see* rights
circumcision *see* female genital
    mutilation, male circumcision
citizenship 67, 68–9; active 59–61;
    duties 206; *see also* rights
Cleveland sexual abuse cases 187
communitarianism 18–19, 66–7,
    161–2
community 29–30, 203, 206–7
complexity 159–63
consent: to medical treatment 113;
    psychoanalysis and 147; sexuality,
    power and 28–9, 179–80, 191–5;
    retrospective 106
contractualism 61–4, 69
courts: children's 54–5, 57–8,
    160–1; and children's conflicting
    wishes 171–2; giving evidence in

148; therapeutic and courtrooms
    in the mind 168–73; wardship
    powers 40
crisis of childhood 25, 127–32
culpability 55, 217–18
culture 5; cultural pluralism 101–2;
    cultural sensitivity 93–6, 97;
    cultural variance and defining
    child abuse 21, 84–5;
    psychoanalysis and cultural issues
    148–50; Western humanism and
    other cultures 96–9

definitions 19–22; child abuse
    19–21, 74–89
delinquency 55, 123; *see also* juvenile
    offenders
dependence 37, 123–5, 131;
    autonomy, agency and 132–3
development: bio-social 191;
    ideology of 221; moral 152;
    optimal 86
dialogic community 18, 65–6, 67
dialogic justice 168–9
disability 217; psychoanalysts and
    parents with 149–50; special
    educational needs 31–2, 221, 222
disruptive behaviour 31–2, 212–29
distributional justice 18–19, 53–73

eating disorders 115, 150–1
education: behavioural difficulties
    31–2, 212–29; moral campaigns
    39, 43–4, 45–6, 54; National
    Curriculum 226;
    problematization of behaviour
    214–15; school's appeal
    committees 215–16, 217; special
    needs assessment 222
Education Act 1870 45
Education Act 1996 221
Education Act 1997 212, 218–19,
    226 ·
Education (Provision of Meals) Act
    1906 45
elementary schools 45
emotional abuse 80
employment legislation 37–8

Milton Keynes UK
Ingram Content Group UK Ltd.
UKHW040012071024
449327UK00011B/197